EDUCATION CENTRE LIBRARY
FURNESS GENERAL HOSPITAL
BARROW-IN-FURNESS

D1080003

22.83

Handbook of
Colposcopy

Handbook of Colposcopy

Edited by

David Luesley, Mahmood Shafi and Joe Jordan

A member of the Hodder Headline Group
LONDON

First published in Great Britain in 1996 by Chapman & Hall
Reprinted in 2000 by
Arnold, a member of the Hodder Headline Group,
338 Euston Road, London NW1 3BH

http://www.arnoldpublishers.com

Co-published in the USA by
Oxford University Press Inc.,
198 Madison Avenue, New York, NY10016
Oxford is a registered trademark of Oxford University Press

©1996 Chapman & Hall, 1999 Arnold

SMC

618.4
LUE

All rights reserved. No part of this publication may be reproduced or
transmitted in any form or by any means, electronically or mechanically,
including photocopying, recording or any information storage or retrieval
system, without either prior permission in writing from the publisher or a
licence permitting restricted copying. In the United Kingdom such licences
are issued by the Copyright Licensing Agency: 90 Tottenham Court Road,
London W1P 0LP.

Whilst the advice and information in this book are believed to be true and
accurate at the date of going to press, neither the authors nor the publisher
can accept any legal responsibility or liability for any errors or omissions
that may be made. In particular (but without limiting the generality of the
preceding disclaimer) every effort has been made to check drug dosages;
however, it is still possible that errors have been missed. Furthermore,
dosage schedules are constantly being revised and new side-effects
recognized. For these reasons the reader is strongly urged to consult the
drug companies' printed instructions before administering any of the drugs
recommended in this book.

British Library Cataloguing in Publication Data
A catalogue record for this book is available from the British Library

Library of Congress Cataloging-in-Publication Data
A catalog record for this book is available from the Library of Congress

ISBN 0 412 71550 3

2 3 4 5 6 7 8 9 10

Typeset in 10 on 12pt Times by West Key Ltd., Falmouth, Cornwall
Printed and bound by the Athenaeum Press, Gateshead

What do you think about this book? Or any other Arnold title?
Please send your comments to feedback.arnold@hodder.co.uk

Contents

Contributors

Dr M.C Anderson
Reader in Gynaecological Pathology, Department of Histopathology, Queen's Medical Centre, Clifton Boulevard, Nottingham NG7 2UH

Dr J. Cordiner
Consultant Obstetrician and Gynaecologist, Queen Mother's Hospital, Yorkhill, Glasgow G3 8SH and Western Infirmary, Glasgow G11 6NT

Dr G.P. Downey
56 Chantry Road, Moseley, Birmingham, B13 8DJ

Dr I.D. Duncan
Reader in Obstetrics and Gynaecology, Ninewells Hospital and Medical School, Dundee, DD1 9SY

Mr D.A. Hicks
Consultant Physician in GU Medicine, Department of Genitourinary Medicine, Royal Hallamshire Hospital, Glossop Road, Sheffield S10 2JF

Mr J.A. Jordan
Director, Birmingham Maternity Hospital, Queen Elizabeth Medical Centre, Metchley Road, Edgbaston, Birmingham B18 7QH

Professor H. Kitchener
Consultant Gynaecologist, Aberdeen Royal Infirmary, Foresterhill, Aberdeen AB9 2ZB and Professor of Obstetrics and Gynaecology, St Mary's Hospital, Manchester

Mr F.G. Lawton
Consultant Gynaecologist, Department of Obstetrics and Gynaecology, King's College Hospital, Denmark Hill, London SE5 8RX

Mr D. M. Luesley
Reader in Gynaecological Oncology, Directorate of Obstetrics and Gynaecology, City Hospital NHS Trust, Dudley Road, Birmingham B18 7QH

Dr J. Murphy
Blackrock Clinic, Rock Road, Co. Dublin, EIRE

Mr C. W. E. Redman
Consultant Obstetrician and Gynaecologist, Academic Department of Obstetrics and Gynaecology, North Staffordshire Hospital NHS Trust, Newcastle Road, Stoke-on-Trent ST4 6QG

Dr T. P. Rollason
Consultant Histopathologist, Department of Pathology, Birmingham Maternity Hospital, Edgbaston, Birmingham B15 2TG

Mr M. I. Shafi
Senior Lecturer, Directorate of Obstetrics and Gynaecology, City Hospital NHS Trust, Dudley Road, Birmingham B18 7QH

Mr P. Walker
Consultant Gynaecologist, The Royal Free Hospital, Pond St, London NW3

Mr D. R. Williams
Department of Academic Gynaecology, Birmingham Women's Hospital, Edgbaston, Birmingham B15 2TG

Abbreviations

AIS	Adenocarcinoma-*in-situ*
ASCUS	Atypical squamous cells of uncertain significance
AW	Acetowhite
BNA	Borderline nuclear abnormalities
BSCC	British Society of Cervical Cytology
BSCCP	British Society of Colposcopy and Cervical Pathology
cGIN	Cervical glandular intraepithelial neoplasia
CIN	Cervical intraepithelial neoplasia
CTZ	Congenital transformation zone
DES	Diethylstilboestrol
DLE	Diathermy loop excision
ECC	Endocervical curettage
ESI	Early stormal invasion (now more correctly stage la1 cancer)
FHSA	Family Health Service Authority
FIGO	International Federation of Obstetrics and Gynecology
GUM	Genitourinary medicine
HPV	Human papillomavirus
HSV	Herpes simplex virus
IFCPC	International Society of Cervical Pathology and Colposcopy
K	Koilocytes or koilocytosis
LEEP	Loop electrosurgical excisional procedure
LLETZ	Large loop excision of the transformation zone
MIN	Multifocal intraepithelial neoplasia
NAC	National Association of Cytologists
NCN	National Co-ordinating Network
NHSCSP	National Health Service Cervical Screening Programme
PIN	Perineal intraepithelial neoplasia
RCOG	Royal College of Obstetricians and Gynaecologists
SCJ	Squamocolumnar junction

TV	*Trichomonas vaginalis*
TZ	Transformation zone
ValN	Vaginal intraepithelial neoplasia
VIN	Vulvar intraepithelial neoplasia

The normal anatomy and histology of the cervix

T. P. Rollason

GROSS ANATOMY

The cervix is the most caudal portion of the uterus and protrudes into the upper vagina. It measures 2.5–3 cm in length in the adult multigravida and makes up one-third to one-half of the length of the uterus. The cervix is demarcated from the uterine corpus by a fibromuscular junction termed the internal os and the endocervical canal opens into the vaginal vault at the external os. The vagina is fused circumferentially to the cervix, dividing it into an upper, supravaginal and a lower, vaginal portion. These portions are of approximately the same length. As the uterus is normally anteverted the cervix is usually angled downward and backward. The shape of the cervix is highly variable. The nulliparous cervix has a circular external os and a diameter of approximately 2.0–2.5 cm. The multiparous cervix is larger and more protruding and has a transverse, slit-like external os. The reflections of the vaginal epithelium around the sides of the cervix constitute the vaginal fornices. The vaginal portion of the cervix (portio vaginalis) is divided into anterior and posterior lips; the anterior is shorter and projects lower than the posterior. Both cervical lips are normally in contact with the posterior vaginal wall.

The cervical canal connects the uterine isthmus (internal os) with the external os. This is an elliptical cavity showing longitudinal ridges (plicae palmatae) composed of epithelium and connective tissue. The canal has a

Handbook of Colposcopy, edited by David Luesley, Mahmood Shafi and Joe Jordan. Published in 1996 by Chapman & Hall, London. ISBN 0 412 71550 3

maximum diameter of approximately 7–8 mm. It is approximately 3 cm long and is flattened antero-posteriorly.

The cervical stroma is made up of fibrous, muscular and elastic tissue. Fibrous tissue predominates, with smooth muscle located mainly in the endocervix and increasing in relative proportion as the internal os is approached. At the isthmus smooth muscle and fibrous tissue are present in approximately equal proportions and in concentric arrangement, making up a functional sphincter.

Congenital abnormalities of the cervix usually result from abnormal development and fusion of the Müllerian ducts and are usually therefore seen in association with uterine body maldevelopment.

HISTOLOGY

'Original' (native) squamous epithelium

The vaginal portion of the cervix (ectocervix) is lined by stratified squamous epithelium, which in its normal state is not keratinized on light microscopy. This epithelium is replenished by proliferation of basal cells every 4–5 days during reproductive life. Maturation may be accelerated by oestrogens and inhibited, at the mid-zone of the epithelium, by progestagens. In adult life this epithelium is fully mature and glycogen-laden due to oestrogenic stimulation. In postmenopausal women the epithelium undergoes atrophy, with thinning, loss of differentiation and loss of glycogen; the whole epithelium then appears to consist of basal and parabasal-type cells. In the prepubertal female the epithelium is of similar appearance to that of the postmenopausal woman. During pregnancy superficial maturation is lost under the influence of elevated progesterone.

It is usual to divide the ectocervical epithelium into three zones; basal; mid-zone and superficial (Fig. 1.1). The basal zone is composed of one or two layers of cylindrical or elliptical cells approximately 10 nm in diameter. These have scant cytoplasm and nuclei orientated perpendicular to the underlying

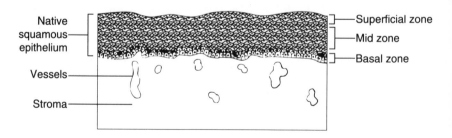

Fig. 1.1 Ectocervical squamous epithelium.

basal lamina (basal membrane). The cells of this layer are actively dividing. The lower few layers of the mid-zone contain larger cells than the basal layer with more cytoplasm, often termed parabasal cells. In normal epithelium mitoses are seen in these cells as well as the basal layer but with less frequency. Glycogen synthesis occurs in this layer. The upper mid-zone or intermediate cell zone is composed of non-dividing, glycogen-rich cells which show a gradual increase in cytoplasm with increasing height. The overall pattern of this zone is often termed 'basket-weave'. The cells of the superficial zone show flattening and an overall cell diameter of approximately 50 nm. The nuclei are small and pyknotic and the cytoplasm glycogen-rich and eosinophilic. The epithelial surface is cornified and on electron microscopy a complex surface pattern of microridges is present; these are believed to help prevent trauma to the underlying layers and stop infective agents entering the deep epithelium. Under some exogenous stimuli keratinization occurs above the superficial cells; this is represented by a dense, eosinophilic layer of variable thickness.

The atrophic epithelium of postmenopausal women shows little or no surface epithelial maturation and absent or sparse stromal papillae (rete pegs are not normally seen even in the mature cervix).

'Original' (native) columnar epithelium

The endocervical columnar epithelium is composed of a single layer of mucin-secreting, columnar cells. These cells have basally placed, round or oval nuclei and uniform, slightly granular cytoplasm filled with mucin droplets (Müllerian mucinous epithelium). The relative proportions of different mucins vary with the menstrual cycle. These changes in the histochemical composition of the mucins are reflected in the actual physical consistency of the mucus; at midcycle it is more watery, less viscous and more abundant than at other times in the cycle and it shows the capacity for 'ferning' in smears. Occasional non-secretory cells with cilia are present, resembling tubal or endometrial ciliated cells; these probably play a role in mucin movement. On two-dimensional sections the endocervix appears to show surface epithelium and variably spaced, underlying tubular elements.

While the endocervical surface epithelium is often referred to as a mucosa and the tubular elements as glands, neither is actually true. The surface epithelium and epithelium of the underlying structures have no associated submucosa and are a simple epithelium, not a mucosal surface. The endocervical 'glands' are actually deep, cleft-like infoldings of the surface epithelium with numerous blind secondary outpouchings (Fig. 1.2). The epithelium of the crypts is identical to that of the surface whereas true glands have different epithelium in their ductal elements to that in their secretory portions. Although crypts have been stated to occasionally be more than 1 cm deep, the maximum depth in well orientated sections is closer to 8 mm (mean 3.4 mm). It is usually said that the endocervical epithelium has an origin in

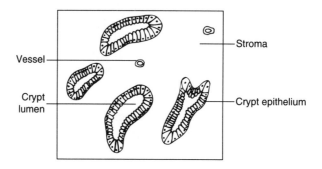

Fig. 1.2 Endocervical crypts.

the subcolumnar reserve cells and that mitoses are not seen in the columnar epithelium in normal conditions.

The endocervical epithelium, as well as crypt infolding, also shows coarse mounds or cushions called rugae, which are present on both lips of the cervix. This rugal pattern fuses with the longitudinal 'arbor vitae' in the canal (the plicae palmatae previously referred to). There is a further fine grouping of folds to produce pendulous areas resembling bunches of grapes.

Squamous metaplasia and the transformation zone

The squamocolumnar junction (SCJ) of the cervix is the point at which the endocervical columnar epithelium meets the ectocervical stratified squamous epithelium (Fig. 1.3). This junction is not at a fixed point on the cervix throughout life. The understanding of the changes that occur at the SCJ throughout life is fundamental to an understanding of the processes leading up to tumour formation in the cervix.

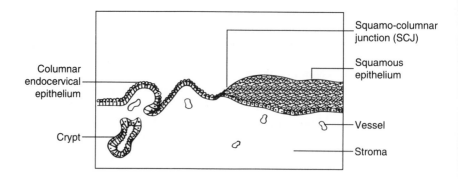

Fig. 1.3 The 'original' squamocolumnar junction.

Before puberty, the SCJ is usually accepted to be located at, or close to, the external os of the cervix. This point is often called the 'original' SCJ. The junction is a sharp one. Under the influence of increasing ovarian hormones at puberty there is an increase in the size of both the corpus and cervix. This leads to eversion of the cervix which is more marked anteriorly and posteriorly than laterally and usually most extensive on the anterior lip. The endocervical epithelium then comes to lie on the vaginal portion of the cervix. This endocervical epithelium appears red and rough and is often clinically termed an erosion (incorrect, as no ulceration is present) or an ectopy (ectropion). This zone of eversion is most extensive in women under 20 years of age and following the first pregnancy. The everted zone, particularly when extensive, commonly takes on a papillary pattern with a chronic inflammatory cell infiltrate in the stromal cores of the papillae. This pattern is often termed papillary cervicitis but is a physiological change, not a true cervicitis.

The zone of eversion is exposed to the acidic environment of the vagina and it appears to be predominantly this stimulus that leads to the series of changes which follow and culminate in replacement of the everted endocervical epithelium by more resilient squamous epithelium. Two major mechanisms have in the past been favoured: the first is direct ingrowth of the adjacent squamous epithelium of the portio. Tongues of squamous epithelium grow beneath the adjacent columnar epithelium and expand between the endocervical mucinous cells and the basement membrane. The endocervical cells are gradually displaced upwards, degenerate and are sloughed. It is unclear how important a role this mechanism has. Certainly this process cannot explain the occasional presence of isolated foci of squamous metaplasia within the endocervical canal.

The second process is usually called squamous metaplasia but the process is not a truly metaplastic one, metaplasia being the replacement of one adult, differentiated epithelium by another of different type. In the first part of the process small, non-differentiated, cuboidal reserve cells, with a high nucleo–cytoplasmic ratio, appear beneath the columnar epithelium. These usually appear first on the upper, more exposed parts of the villous outgrowths and superficial crypts. The reserve cells proliferate to produce a layer several cells thick (reserve cell hyperplasia). At this stage the columnar cells remain as a complete or incomplete surface layer. These multilayered reserve cells then begin differentiation to clearly squamous cells with increasing amounts of eosinophilic cytoplasm, but without surface maturation and with little intracellular glycogen and a now incomplete persisting surface columnar cell layer (incomplete or immature squamous metaplasia) (Fig. 1.4). Finally all the surface columnar cells are shed or degenerate and the squamous epithelium fully matures. There is therefore now a new squamocolumnar junction (the 'physiological' or 'functional' SCJ). The zone where columnar epithelium has been converted to squamous is termed the 'transformation zone' (Fig. 1.5).

Viewed at the end of the process of metaplasia, the transformation zone epithelium may be indistinguishable from the native ectocervical epithelium.

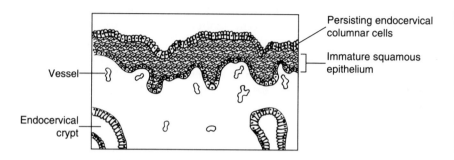

Fig. 1.4 Immature squamous metaplasia.

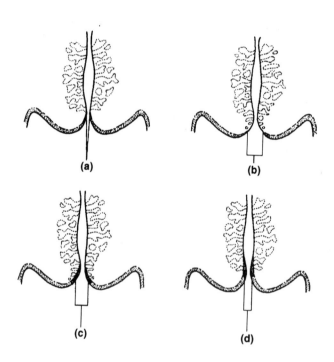

Fig. 1.5 Relative changes in the position of the squamocolumnar junction and transformation zone as the cervix changes under endocrine influences. **(a)** Original squamocolumnar junction. **(b)** New SCJ. **(c)** Transformation zone (metaplastic squamous epithelium). **(d)** TZ inside canal. (Source: reproduced with permission from Rollason, T. P. (1995) The normal anatomy and histology of the cervix, vagina and vulva, in *Intraepithelial Neoplasia of the Female Lower Genital Tract*, (eds D. Luesley, J. Jordan and Richart), Churchill Livingstone, Edinburgh, ch. 1.)

Apart from hormonal effects and vaginal acidity, other possible causes of metaplasia, and accelerants of the process, include inflammatory damage, chronic irritation, coitus (prostaglandin exposure) and direct trauma.

The process of metaplasia may extend into the shallower underlying crypts for their full depth and eventually obliterate them, but usually the crypts either persist, lined by endocervical epithelium, or are partly lined by squamous cells. That surface epithelium is metaplastic may therefore be deduced from the presence of underlying crypts, as there is very little overlapping of crypts by 'original' squamous surface cells. The openings of the crypts may still be evident on the cervical surface of the transformation zone but the squamous proliferation may lead to their blockage; this produces the very common 'Nabothian follicles'. These are in reality mucus retention cysts of the crypts due to continued mucin production, with cystic dilatation related to lack of mucin drainage. The cysts may rupture leading to a local macrophage response, sometimes with associated inflammation and fibrosis. If the crypts become completely separated from the surface epithelium after the crypt epithelium has undergone replacement by squamous cells then a squamous inclusion cyst may develop.

While, as previously indicated, cervical eversion and thus squamous metaplasia are most marked during adolescence and pregnancy the process continues throughout adult life and all stages of the processes described above are commonly seen in cervical biopsy specimens. After the menopause the shrinkage of the cervical stroma causes 'retraction' of the SCJ into the endocervical canal. The process of squamous metaplasia is not a reversible one and the canal is then lined in its lower portion by squamous epithelium.

THE CONGENITAL TRANSFORMATION ZONE (CTZ)

The CTZ is essentially a zone where endocervical epithelium has undergone squamous metaplasia in late intrauterine or early extrauterine life. It appears to be related to metaplasia in a zone of endocervical epithelium which passed on to the portio under the influence of maternal oestrogen and was replaced by squamous epithelium when the oestrogenic stimulus declined. Alternatively, it may be that the CTZ is formed in a similar manner to essentially identical zones seen in DES exposed women, i.e. due to incomplete conversion of the early cuboidal epithelium of the vaginal angle at the upper (uterine) end to squamous epithelium, followed by gradual squamous replacement in late intrauterine and extrauterine life.

The histological features of the CTZ in a typical case are: a thinned epithelium with shallow, fine (but blunt-ended) epithelial downgrowths; low or absent epithelial glycogen; and a very fine layer of surface keratinization (Fig. 1.6).

The epithelium gives the impression of being immature in its lower half, but

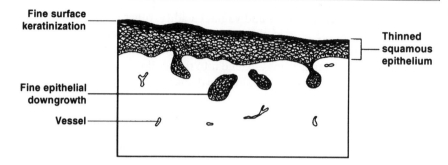

Fig. 1.6 The congenital transformation zone.

maturing abnormally rapidly to keratinization over a few cell layers. The junction with the 'normal' ectocervical squamous epithelium is usually tangential but sharp and, when seen in the adult, the CTZ is usually separated from the SCJ by a zone of more typical 'adult'-type squamous metaplasia. The low glycogen, thin epithelium, etc. may lead to a mistaken colposcopic impression of CIN.

CERVICAL CHANGES DURING PREGNANCY

Under the stimulus of gestational hormones the cervix softens and enlarges. This is due to increased vascularity and stromal oedema. Acute inflammatory changes are also commonly seen in the superficial stroma. In late pregnancy there is accumulation of large amounts of extracellular glycoprotein and collagen disruption leading to further softening, facilitating dilatation, etc. in labour. Decidualization of the stroma under progestational effects is common in the superficial stroma. It may be patchy or diffuse and affects both endo- and ectocervix. Some degree of decidualization occurs in more than one-third of pregnant women and takes some weeks to disappear after delivery.

Macroscopically, deciduous foci appear as raised, vascular nodules and colposcopically they may closely resemble invasive carcinoma. Very occasionally foci of decidualization may be seen in the absence of pregnancy or obvious endometriosis, usually in association with progestagen therapy.

As indicated previously, very extensive zones of cervical 'erosion' are classically seen in pregnancy and immature metaplasia and reserve cell hyperplasia are extensive. This is most striking in primigravidae. There are probably two major processes underlying the epithelial changes seen. The first is the eversion of the endocervical canal epithelium, and the second is gaping of the os. These changes are more marked in the first pregnancy and tend to occur later in pregnancy in multiparous women.

LEARNING POINTS

1. **Ectocervical epithelium** is stratified squamous epithelium. It repopulates every 5 days. Oestrogen shortens the repopulation time. In the elderly atrophy occurs and differentiation is reduced, making cytological and histological interpretation difficult.

2. **Endocervical epithelium** is a columnar, mucinous Müllerian epithelium. Branching epithelial downgrowths are present, producing crypts, These are not true glands.

3. **The squamocolumnar junction (SCJ)** is the border between the squamous ectocervical epithelium and the endocervical columnar epithelium. The 'original' SCJ is where the 'native' epithelium met the endocervical epithelium in childhood. The 'physiological' SCJ is where the SCJ is seen after the effects of endogenous and exogenous hormones, pregnancy, etc.

4. **The transformation zone** is the area where the native endocervical epithelium has been converted to squamous epithelium. This new squamous epithelium covers endocervical crypts and the crypts' openings may be still present or the crypts represented by spherical surface humps 2–4 mm in diameter. Nabothian follicles are mucus retention cysts formed by the blockage of the crypt neck by the squamous overgrowth.

5. **Squamous metaplasia** is the alteration of the endocervical columnar epithelium into squamous epithelium. It occurs via a stage of undifferentiated reserve cell growth (reserve cell hyperplasia) followed by squamous differentiation. Immature metaplasia is the stage at which there is squamous replacement but with retention of surface endocervical columnar cells. Laser therapy, trauma, etc. speeds up the metaplastic process.

6. **Congenital transformation zone (CTZ)**: In intrauterine or early postuterine life changes in hormonal profile lead to the formation of a limited transformation zone of different pattern to that in the adult. This persists into adult life and shows low epithelial glycogen content, fine surface keratinization and fine epithelial downgrowths.

7. **Ectopy or erosion**: In reproductive life columnar epithelium is seen on the ectocervical surface to some extent; this is often clinically referred to as an ectopy or erosion. It is usually more extensive on the anterior lip. The formation of such endocervical-lined zones is stimulated by oestrogens, progestagens and, particularly, pregnancy, after which they may persist for some years. Papillary cervicitis (papillary ectropion) is simply a variant of this pattern.

8. **Decidualization** occurs in pregnancy and both focal and diffuse decidualization of the cervical stroma may occur. This change is associated with increased vascularization and oedema and may be mistaken clinically for malignancy.

MCQS

1. The ectocervical native epithelium is:
    a. Of columnar mucinous type
    b. Sensitive to hormone effects
    c. Of multilayered squamous type
    d. Commonly ulcerated
    e. Very fragile in comparison to the endocervical epithelium

2. The 'physiological' SCJ:
    a. Is where the squamous and endocervical epithelium met in childhood
    b. Is a fixed point
    c. Moves under the influence of hormones
    d. Is usually within the endocervical canal in the postmenopausal woman
    e. Doesn't exist

3. The transformation zone:
    a. Is where native endocervical epithelium has been converted to squamous epithelium
    b. Persists even into the post-menopausal years
    c. Never has underlying crypts
    d. Can be identified colposcopically by the presence of gland openings

4. Squamous metaplasia is
    a. A pathological process
    b. Brought about by the effect of vaginal acidity
    c. Stimulated by trauma
    d. Caused by Human papillomavirus
    e. Preceded by reserve cell hyperplasia

5. The congenital transformation zone:
    a. Is formed prenatally
    b. Is related to uterine fundal abnormalities
    c. Disappears after the menopause
    d. Is often associated with excess epithelial glycogen production
    e. Is invisible colposcopically

Cervical cytology

D. R. Williams

HISTORY AND INTRODUCTION

The first illustrations of shed cells from tumours as seen under a microscope were published 150 years ago. These early observations were followed during the next 50 years by descriptions of cells from sputum, urine, cerebrospinal fluid, gastric washings and lymph node aspirates.

Diagnostic cytology of the female genital tract was introduced almost simultaneously by Babes in Bucharest and Papanicolaou in New York, *circa* 1928. However, neither of these seminal observations made any major clinical impact and it was not until Papanicolaou and Traut's later published works on uterine cancer detection in the 1940s that any significant momentum was gained. Today, five decades after the publication of Papanicolaou's atlas, and countless debates on the merits of cytological diagnosis in gynaecology later, it is generally considered that the cervical smear is one of the most effective health tools ever introduced. There is also little doubt that its effectiveness has been considerably improved over the past 20 years by the increasing use of colposcopy. The combination of smear and colposcope provides a very potent weapon in the quest to reduce deaths from cervical cancer.

FALSE-NEGATIVE RESULTS: CAUSES AND IMPLICATIONS FOR SCREENING

The prime concern of a cervical screening programme is to detect those women with significant degrees of precancer and to prevent progression to invasive

Handbook of Colposcopy, edited by David Luesley, Mahmood Shafi and Joe Jordan. Published in 1996 by Chapman & Hall, London. ISBN 0 412 71550 3

disease by destruction or removal of these precursor lesions. The greatest flaw in the detection process is the potential for false-negative results. Unlike diagnostic cytology from other sites, where the test is only part of the overall diagnostic process, in gynaecological screening a negative test may remove the patient from medical care for 3–5 years. False-negative results may occur because of inadequate sampling, incorrect laboratory processing or detection and interpretative errors of the cell samples.

It must be emphasized that cervical cytology is primarily used as a case-finding procedure for squamous precursor lesions (CIN). It does not diagnose invasive lesions reliably. Aggressive tumours can rapidly utilize available blood supply, the presenting surface becoming necrotic and frequently producing an inflammatory exudate only. When sampled, in the absence of relevant symptomatology or suspicion on naked-eye appearance of the cervix at the time of smear-taking, these smears may well be reported as non-specific inflammatory changes only – the classic 'false-negative' smear result. A clinically suspicious cervix must be biopsied regardless of the cytology test result.

The process of screening a cervical smear

It may be worthwhile to underline at this point that cytology is not a precise science, but more an acquired art form. Schenk likens the process of searching for an abnormal cell to 'detecting large cars among smaller cars while flying 1000 metres high in an area 230 kilometres in length and 720 metres broad within five minutes at a velocity of twice the speed of sound'. Primary screeners rely heavily on experience for building up a mental database of case recognition features. This database is reinforced by comparisons of cytological predictions *versus* final histological outcome. The frequency of encountering these features is a major factor in adding weight to likelihood of underlying pathology. This cannot be 'taught' easily with conventional demonstration/response training routines, as intensive exposure to archival rarities frequently results in overcalling and a subsequent lack of trust by the clinical team. So, while practical exposure to common cytological categories of cervical disease is essential – and with experience reliably uniform – cytological encounters with rare disease states are frequently overlooked, screening omissions being revealed with clinical presentation and subsequent biopsy. However, careful observation and audit of practice with continuing input from accumulated knowledge should maintain reasonable accuracy of detection and minimize false negatives (sensitivity) and false positives (specificity).

Recently, the problem of screener performance has been addressed by the adoption of rapid rescreening of all negative smears, the proscription of sensible targets and standards for service provision, and the participation in external quality assurance schemes by all laboratories working in the NHS Cervical Screening Programme.

HOW TO TAKE AND PREPARE SMEARS

The accuracy of the cytological examination of a cervical smear depends predominantly on the quality of the material collected and the preparation and staining thereafter. Doctors or nurses taking the smear must be fully aware of the purpose and principles of the screening programme, and should ideally have attended a recommended course of instruction in smear-taking and counselling.

Instruments for taking a smear

There are currently a variety of samplers available for smear-taking both from the cervix and the endocervical canal, although it must be emphasized that endocervical brush sampling is not a part of routine screening, but is useful in smears post-treatment or perhaps when an endocervical lesion is suspected. If other non-standard techniques are employed then this should be clearly stated on the request form. Not all laboratories are experienced in the differing appearances from these samplers and high pick-up of minor cytological abnormalities, poor discrimination between reactive and neoplastic appearances, and a high number of inadequate samples may follow (Fig. 2.1).

Ayre and Aylesbury spatulas

Most smears will be taken with a standard Ayres spatula or the modified Aylesbury version. In any event, the most important feature is in the application of the sampler and not the particular shape or design.

The aim of the smear is to sample the whole of the transformation zone (TZ), which should be achieved with a full 360° sweep, first clockwise then anticlockwise, with the blade of the spatula firmly applied to the cervix. If bleeding occurs on the first sweep, the spatula should be withdrawn and the cells thus obtained spread and fixed immediately.

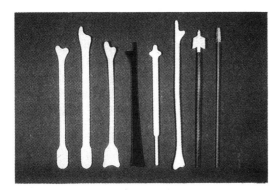

Fig. 2.1 Commercially available sampling devices.

If the transformation zone is on the outer aspect of the ectocervix, this should be sampled, after the usual rotational cell collection, with firm diagonal sweeps encompassing the apparent squamocolumnar junction.

If there is blood or purulent mucus covering the os, this should be gently pushed side by the sampler before the smear is taken. Generalized swabbing is not recommended as diagnostic cells may be lost.

Cervex brush

The technique using the Cervex brush is similar, but the bristles are 'D-shaped' and their cutting edge is designed to work in a clockwise fashion. With the long bristles introduced into the os, the brush should be rotated clockwise five times, with the short bristles applied more closely to the ectocervix.

Cytobrush, Axibrush, etc. endocervical brush samplers

Endocervical samples should always be paired with ectocervical smears to achieve adequate TZ sampling. The endocervical brush should be introduced into the canal until only the last row of bristles is just visible at the external os, and then rotated through 180° only. If the brush head is pushed too far into the canal, endometrial sampling may occur, causing possible confusion to the cytologist.

Owing to the tendency of this device to cause bleeding, ectocervical sampling should always precede endocervical collection.

Making the slide

The aim is to produce an even, thin film across the whole surface of the glass slide, which should be clearly prelabelled with patient surname and date of birth in pencil on the frosted end.

Both sides of the sampler should be spread swiftly and deliberately on to the slide on the same side as the frosted label. Straight, neat strokes are preferred.

If an endocervical brush sample is taken the cells should be rolled on to the slide with a firm, rolling motion. Ecto- and endocervical samples taken at the same visit may be spread on a single slide, but if this is done the samples must be spread side by side and not superimposed. The endocervical brush sample should be spread second as it has a greater tendency to air-dry than spatula-collected samples, and the laboratory must be informed so that a longer coverslip may be used.

Fixation

Once the cells are removed they must be preserved immediately. Alcohol is the fixative of choice and is usually supplied in small pots, dropper bottles or aerosol sprays. Fixation must be within 30 seconds of spreading, as air-drying causes loss of nuclear detail, making the smear unreadable.

JUDGING THE ACCURACY OF THE SMEAR

It is the responsibility of the smear-taker to ensure that the whole of the TZ has been adequately sampled. It is not possible for the laboratory to be certain that the full circumference of the cervix has been sampled whatever the cellularity or cell content of the smear. A smear taken from half the cervix would look the same as one from the whole circumference.

The laboratory should provide information on the cervical smear report as to whether or not there are indicators of probable TZ sampling, based on the presence of immature metaplastic squamous and/or endocervical cells, but this is primarily for local quality assurance purposes and cannot guarantee absolute smear adequacy. It must be remembered that there are no reliable indicators of TZ sampling in atrophic smears.

SMEAR REPORTS

Negative and inflammatory smears

No smear should be reported as negative unless it has a sufficient quantity of squamous cells, taking into account the woman's age and hormonal status.

A wide range of benign reactive changes may be seen in cervical cells, particularly in metaplastic cells. Inflammation of the cervix is common, but the epithelial cell changes associated with acute and chronic inflammation and repair processes can usually be distinguished from neoplasia with experience.

Trichomonas vaginalis, Candida, Actinomyces-like organisms, bacteria and Herpes simplex cytopathic effect may all be present in routine smears. These features should be reported as negative with a normal recommendation for recall. There is no indication for the recommendation of an early repeat in such smears just because they harbour an infection and minor degrees of inflammatory reaction. If dyskaryosis has been eliminated, these changes should be passed without comment.

Inadequate smears

Smears are reported as inadequate in the following circumstances:

1. The smear is too thick, but the presence of blood and/or leukocytes in large numbers with or without any recognizable treatable condition (*Trichomonas vaginalis*, Herpes simplex, *Candida, Actinomyces*, atrophy)

does not necessarily make a smear inadequate, providing the material is adequately fixed, well spread and extra care is taken in examining the material.

2. The smear contains too few cells for an opinion, bearing in mind that the atrophic cervix will yield very few cells and that drying artefacts may be commonly encountered as a consequence.

3. Smears consist entirely of endocervical cells, a particular consequence of endocervical sampling.

4. Smears are poorly fixed or air-dried to the degree that assessment is impossible.

An acceptable range of smears falling within this category would be between 5% and 9%.

Borderline nuclear abnormalities

Inevitably, as with any subjective process, there will be grey areas when cellular changes differentiating benign atypia from early dyskaryosis are not cut-and-dried. The British Society of Cervical Cytology (BSCC) introduced the term 'borderline nuclear abnormalities' (BNA) to be used in such cases, while the international cytological community favours the acronyms ASCUS (atypical squamous cells of undetermined significance), and AGUS (atypical glandular cells of undetermined significance).

There are two broad situations when the 'borderline' category is invoked. The commonest, and often least clinically significant, is when drawing the fine diagnostic line between HPV change and mild dyskaryosis. The second situation covers a diverse group of conditions in which it may be difficult to distinguish benign, reactive or reparative changes from significant degrees of dyskaryosis, or even invasive cancer on occasions.

Endocervical cells may also exhibit equivocal nuclear changes, which require considerable diagnostic experience and skill to determine their significance. Great caution should be exercised in dealing with this category, with repeat smears recommended after a maximum of 6 months and no more than once before colposcopic referral. Failure to observe this simple advice has frequently led to the subsequent development of an advanced invasive endocervical cancer, presenting following the 'minimally abnormal endocervical' index smear inadequately followed up or ignored. Unfortunately, this situation is almost as well known to the legal profession as to our own of late.

An achievable standard range for borderline and mildly dyskaryotic smears is $5.5 \pm 1.5\%$.

Dyskaryosis

Dyskaryosis is the cytological nuclear change associated with a histological diagnosis of CIN. Correlation of mild, moderate and severe dyskaryosis with

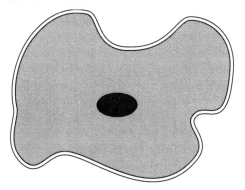

Fig. 2.2 Diagrammatic representation of a normal squamous cell as determined by the relationship between nuclear and cytoplasmic area.

CIN 1, 2, and 3 is not exact, but moderate dyskaryosis or worse usually indicates at least underlying CIN 2 (Figs 2.2, 2.3). Mild dyskaryosis usually corresponds with CIN 1 but there may be small areas of CIN 2 or 3 on the same cervix. Thus the cytological degree of dyskaryosis should be taken to indicate the minimum degree of CIN. The terminology and definitions of CIN are described in more detail in Chapter 3.

Dyskaryosis is frequently associated with Human papillomavirus (HPV) change, but the presence of HPV change should not affect the recommendations for management, which should only be based on the degree of dyskaryosis.

Mild dyskaryosis should be an indication for referral on its second occurrence.

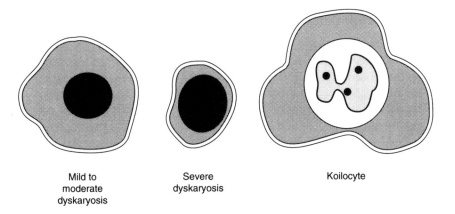

Mild to moderate dyskaryosis

Severe dyskaryosis

Koilocyte

Fig. 2.3 Diagrammatic representation of dyskaryotic cells demonstrating an increased nuclear/cytoplasmic ratio.

Moderate dyskaryosis is very subjective and impossible to define. Its severity lies somewhere between mild and severe dyskaryosis! Dyskaryotic cells that are difficult to grade (usually because of their scarcity in the smear) will usually be coded and managed as for moderate dyskaryosis. This is particularly important in recurrence of CIN after treatment, when abnormal cells may be few. HPV changes will also confound opinion.

Severe dyskaryosis is usually seen in cells with abnormal cytoplasmic maturation and a high nuclear/cytoplasmic ratio; however, it may occur with intracytoplasmic keratinization, which should not be mistaken for HPV change. Moderate (including ungraded) dyskaryosis, severe dyskaryosis, ?invasive and ?glandular neoplasia are all indications for gynaecological referral on their first occurrence.

Smears showing severe dyskaryosis in which there is tumour diathesis may be reported as suggesting cytological evidence of invasion.

The achievable standard range for moderate/severe dyskaryosis is $1.6 \pm 0.4\%$

BSCC TERMINOLOGY – EXTRACTS FROM BSCC PUBLICATIONS

'It is axiomatic that cytology reports are not only scientifically accurate but also easily understood so that the patient receives appropriate management and advice.'

'The cytology report on abnormal findings should consist of a precise description of cells in precisely defined and generally accepted cytological terms. This may be followed, if appropriate, by a prediction of the histological condition based on the overall picture, and should include a recommendation for the further management of the patient. For this reason the smear report is considered a medical consultation.'

'When a prediction of histology is included as a supplementary statement to a description of the cytology, use of the terminology cervical intra-epithelial neoplasia (CIN) is preferred: it has the advantage of relating the histological report more clearly to the prognosis and management than the artificial separation implied by classification into dysplasia and carcinoma *in situ*. Caution is advised however in the firm prediction of CIN 3 because the cytologist cannot reliably exclude a microinvasive or invasive lesion.'

The histological prediction is more accurately recorded on the National Cytology Form, HMR101/5 (1982), where severe dysplasia or carcinoma *in situ* (CIN 3), or carcinoma *in situ* (CIN 3) or ?invasive carcinoma are the alternatives provided.

SCREENING PROGRAMME GUIDELINES

The policy on the National Cervical Screening Programme is set out in Health Service Guidelines (HSG(93)41) in conjunction with recent NHS reforms and *The Health of the Nation* targets.

The White Paper *The Health of the Nation* set a national target to reduce the mortality of cervical cancer by at least 20% by the year 2000 (from 15/100 000 population in 1986 to no more than 12/100 000, directly standardized against European population). This reduction should be achieved through regular screening of women aged 20–64 to enable prompt treatment of conditions that otherwise would have a significant risk of development into cervical cancer.

Health authorities should aim to achieve and maintain at least 80% coverage, in line with the GP target payment scheme, which provides for higher and lower payments when 80% and 50% of women aged 20–64 years registered with a practice have been screened in the previous 5.5 years.

It is essential that all abnormal smears are followed up. Guidelines on fail-safe mechanisms for the follow-up of cervical smears are published by the NHS Cervical Screening Programme National Co-ordinating Network (ed. I. D. Duncan, Oxford, 1992).

In summary the objectives of the NHSCSP are set out below.

1. To identify and invite eligible women for a cervical smear.
2. To cover the population with effective and acceptable testing.
3. To give women information about the benefits and limitations of the cervical smear test.
4. To identify cervical intraepithelial neoplasia
5. To follow up all women who are deemed to need further investigation or treatment.
6. To inform women how they can reduce the risk of cervical intraepithelial neoplasia.
7. To provide acceptable and effective investigations and treatment with minimal physical or psychological side effects.
8. To involve women both individually and collectively in the development of the programme.
9. To minimize the adverse effects of screening, namely anxiety and unnecessary investigations.
10. To make the best use of available resources for the benefit of the population at risk.
11. To help those working in the programme to improve their competence and find fulfilment in their work.
12. To evaluate the programme and seek continual improvements in quality.

LEARNING POINTS

1. It should be emphasized to all those working in the National Cervical Screening Programme, including the patient base, that the cervical smear is normally a screening test for asymptomatic women, and that a single normal smear does not rule out invasive cancer. Indeed, false-negative rates may be highest in invasive lesions. Despite this, the smear test may also be used for diagnostic purposes and may also detect other diseases, ranging from infections to other genital tract cancers.

2. The sensitivity, specificity, predictive value and accuracy of cervical cytology is impossible to calculate precisely, because the histological result (the gold standard by which most surveys are compared) is itself subject to observer variation, and biopsy samples may not necessarily be representative of the lesion. Furthermore, outcome of a negative test may not be known for several years after the smear was taken, by which time lesions may have developed *de novo*, progressed or regressed.

3. The anxiety levels in patients requested to return for repeat smears for inadequate or borderline categories is extremely high, and these reports should only be issued after careful deliberation. They should not be driven by fear of litigation or lack of training.

4. The effectiveness of the screening programme essentially depends on the identification and treatment of CIN 3. This is largely achieved by the recognition of severe, and to a lesser extent moderate dyskaryosis on cervical smears.

5. Endocervical abnormalities may be cytologically difficult to interpret, and reports suggesting endocervical lesions, however weighted, should be investigated thoroughly.

MCQS

6. The following statements with regard to cervical smear-taking and reporting are true:
    a. The person taking the smear usually decides if the sample is adequate
    b. A smear report of moderate dyskaryosis should be managed as for mild dyskaryosis
    c. The transformation zone is difficult to sample in postmenopausal patients
    d. Colposcopy is not indicated following a smear report of abnormal endocervical cells
    e. Cervical cytology can reliably detect invasive squamous cell cancer

Cervical intraepithelial neoplasia: terminology and definitions

M. C. Anderson

TERMINOLOGY OF CERVICAL INTRAEPITHELIAL NEOPLASIA

Cervical intraepithelial neoplasia is a spectrum of disease and any divisions that are made within the spectrum are arbitrary and artificial. Attempts at classifying CIN have purported to relate to treatment and thus have depended on the expected natural history of lesions at various points in the spectrum. The most obvious and pragmatic division is between those lesions that are unlikely to progress to invasive carcinoma in the foreseeable future and those lesions that are at risk of progression to invasive disease very soon – the former do not need to be treated immediately and may be observed while the latter require immediate eradication to avoid the risk of cancer developing. It seems clear that abnormalities that lie at the extreme bottom end of the spectrum of CIN may regress and that those at the extreme top end will probably lead to invasive carcinoma but there is a broad band of lesions across the centre of the spectrum whose behaviour is unpredictable. It has been customary, there-fore, to subdivide CIN into three: CIN 1, CIN 2 and CIN 3, a system of terminology that was proposed in 1966. In practice, however, most patholo-gists tend to make a diagnosis of CIN 1 or CIN 3 on most lesions; the diagnosis of CIN 2 is not often made. This may be partly because the extremes of a diagnostic spectrum are easier to be confident about and partly because the

Handbook of Colposcopy, edited by David Luesley, Mahmood Shafi and Joe Jordan. Published in 1996 by Chapman & Hall, London. ISBN 0 412 71550 3

criteria for distinguishing between the grades of CIN, particularly between CIN 1 and CIN 2, are not clearly established. A study of the histological descriptions of the grades of CIN presented below show that most of the criteria used are open to subjective interpretation, and this results in poor consistency of diagnosis, both between observers and even for the same observer at different times.

Within the last few years there has been a trend to move away from the concept of three subdivisions of CIN and to re-establish the more basic notion of two grades. Arguments in favour of this change have been fuelled by studies that have demonstrated the lack of consistency in diagnosis using three grades and by the adoption in the US of the Bethesda System for nomenclature of cytological changes. This system uses the terms 'low-grade squamous intra-epithelial lesion' and 'high-grade squamous intraepithelial lesion' for the subdivisions of the cytological spectrum and there is pressure for the histo-logical classification to follow suit. Thus, low-grade lesions in histology are the equivalent of human papillomavirus infection and CIN 1 while high-grade lesions correspond to CIN 2 and CIN 3. Although this approach appears to fit more rationally with management protocols, it is arguable whether it is justifiable always to link HPV infection with CIN 1 and whether the division between CIN 1 and CIN 2 is the best dividing line between low-grade and high-grade lesions. Furthermore, the distinction between these two grades becomes no easier just because there are only two divisions rather than three. While accepting that there are some good arguments for using a two-tier system of nomenclature for CIN rather than a three-tier system, until it can be demonstrated that the two-tier system in current use in some parts of the world is an advance on the established three-tier system, the latter will continue to be used.

THE HISTOLOGY OF CERVICAL INTRAEPITHELIAL NEOPLASIA

The histological features which are taken into account when assessing CIN are:

1. degree of differentiation;
2. nuclear abnormalities;
3. mitotic activity.

Differentiation

Although the meaning of the terms is slightly different, the words differenti-ation and maturation are very often used synonymously and interchangeably in the cervix. When the cells differentiate and mature towards the surface, stratification is observed. The proportion of the epithelium that shows differentiation is used as a criterion for assessing the degree of CIN. If the cells start to differentiate quite close to the basement membrane so that most of the thickness of the epithelium contains maturing cells, then the degree of CIN is likely to be less than that of an epithelium in which only a narrow zone of surface differentiation is seen.

Nuclear abnormalities

Cervical intraepithelial neoplasia has been shown to have an aneuploid DNA content and it is probably this aneuloid chromosome number that contributes mainly to the nuclear enlargement, hyperchromasia, chromatin clumping and irregularities in size and shape of the nucleus. These features taken together are very important criteria in the diagnosis of CIN and for determining its grade. The degree of nuclear abnormality will very often correlate with the amount of differentiation which is seen; the more severe the nuclear abnormalities, the less is the proportion of epithelium that is differentiated. If the correlation is not present in a particular epithelium, then the degree of nuclear abnormality should be taken as a more reliable guide that the proportion of epithelial thickness showing maturation.

Mitotic activity

The normal squamous epithelium of the cervix shows some mitotic activity, with the mitotic figures being largely confined to the parabasal layers. An increase in the number of mitotic figures is one of the features of CIN and the mitotic figures may be positioned at all levels in the epithelium. The vertical position in the epithelium at which the mitotic figures are found is therefore a useful criterion to be taken into account when deciding on the degree of CIN. Taking all these factors into account, the grades of CIN may be characterized in the following way (Fig. 3.1).

CIN 1

Maturation is present in the upper two-thirds of the epithelium, although slight nuclear atypia persists up to the surface, representing a delay in the nuclear maturation. Nuclear abnormalities are slight and are most marked in the basal third. Mitotic figures are present but not numerous; they are confined to the basal third of the epithelium and abnormal forms are rare.

CIN 2

Maturation is present in the upper half of the epithelium, with nuclear atypia persisting to the surface. Nuclear abnormalities are more marked than in CIN 1 and extend further through the epithelium. Mitotic figures are present and

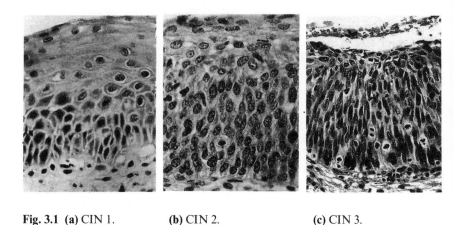

Fig. 3.1 (a) CIN 1. **(b)** CIN 2. **(c)** CIN 3.

are confined to the basal two-thirds of the epithelium. Abnormal forms may be seen.

CIN 3

Maturation may be absent or confined to the superficial third of the epithelium. Nuclear abnormalities are marked throughout most or all of the thickness of the epithelium. Mitotic figures may be numerous and are found at all levels of the epithelium. Abnormal mitoses are frequent. Cervical intraepithelial neoplasia affects both the surface and the crypts. It is essential that crypt involvement is taken into consideration when CIN is being treated, otherwise there is a danger that viable CIN may be left in the depths of the crypts and covered by regenerating stroma and epithelium, perhaps to develop occultly into an invasive carcinoma.

EARLY INVASIVE CARCINOMA

In the earliest recognizable stage of stromal invasion there is a well defined small bud of invasive cells pushing into the stroma, with similar morphology to the CIN 3 from which it has arisen (Fig. 3.2).

As the invasion advances slightly, other morphological features may become apparent. Frequently, the invasive tongues may appear better differentiated than the matrix CIN. There is often a stromal reaction to the invasive tumour, which may be a dense, localized lymphocytic infiltrate or a loosening and apparent oedema of the stroma (condensation of the stroma, the desmoplastic reaction so often seen in other invasive tumours, is rarely present in early invasion in the cervix); often these features are seen together. These three features – better differentiation of the invasive elements, clearing of the

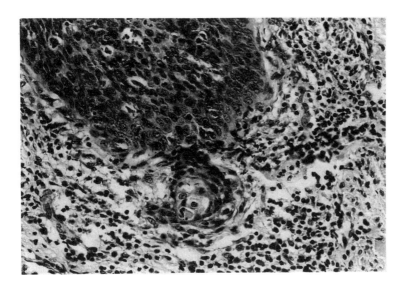

Fig. 3.2 Microinvasive carcinoma. This is a very early stage with a small bud of invasive cells surrounded by a lymphocytic stromal reaction.

stroma and a lymphocytic infiltrate – are changes that can be helpful to the histopathologist in deciding whether early stromal invasion is present or not in ambiguous cases. As the tumour becomes larger and progresses from the individual finger-like processes to a more complex pattern, other morphological features must be taken into account. These are lymphatic channel involvement, the dimension of the tumour and the pattern of growth.

Lymphatic channel involvement

Permeation or invasion of endothelium-lined spaces, which may be either lymphatics or blood vessels, should always be looked for in invasive tumours, however small.

Tumour dimensions

There is general acceptance of the fact that the deeper the tumour invades the worse the prognosis will be and the greater the need for radical treatment. Early invasive carcinomas in the cervix are measured in two dimensions: the first measurement is from the surface (or from the basement membrane of the intraepithelial lesion from which it has arisen, if this can be identified) to the deepest point of invasion and the second measurement is the maximum lateral width of the invasive elements (Fig. 3.3).

The very earliest, finger-like sprouts of invasion usually cannot be

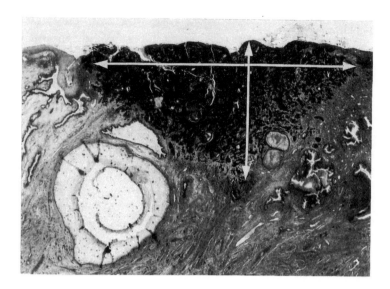

Fig. 3.3 Microinvasive carcinoma. This is a confluent microinvasive lesion showing the two dimensions which are measured.

measured; these are only a fraction of a millimetre deep and are of no significance. It is the larger, measurable but still preclinical lesions that must be measured as accurately as possible and these figures are used to determine the most appropriate treatment (Chapter 13).

Growth pattern

There has been discussion about the value of growth pattern of the early invasive tumour in predicting behaviour and therefore guiding treatment. It has been suggested that a finger-like growth pattern is associated with less aggressive behaviour than a confluent growth pattern, in which multiple islands of tumour infiltrate into the stroma alongside each other. It is likely, however, that the growth pattern depends so much on the size of the invasive tumour that it is not a useful independent variable.

EXAMINATION OF BIOPSY SPECIMENS

The diagnosis of CIN is usually made on either a colposcopically directed punch biopsy, a large loop excision specimen or a conization specimen. Endocervical curettage specimens may also rarely be received. Occasionally a woman with CIN may be treated by hysterectomy.

Colposcopic punch biopsy

During the colposcopic examination saline and acetic acid are applied to the surface of the cervix and it is important that these are applied gently, with a dabbing rather than a rubbing action, so that the fragile epithelium is not dislodged, resulting in a denuded specimen. Biopsies need to be taken after the application of the acetic acid, because it is the application of the acetic acid that identifies where the lesions are, but this does not seem to cause problems or recognizable artefacts. The practice of applying Lugol's iodine before the biopsy is taken should, on the other hand, be strongly discouraged as this solution often causes changes in the superficial layers of the epithelium which can cause confusion and make diagnosis difficult.

Formalin is a perfectly adequate fixative for cervical biopsies of all types. Although Bouin's solution has advantages in the rendering of nuclear detail, the hazards associated with the use of this agent, such as its greater noxiousness and the risk of explosion if it allowed to dry out, outweigh these. The biopsy is bisected transversely with a sharp blade by the pathologist and each half is embedded with the cut surface downwards. Three levels are cut on each half so that six sections are examined from each cervical biopsy received from the colposcopy clinic. An adequate colposcopic biopsy consists of surface epithelium with underlying crypts and stroma. It is important that stromal invasion is excluded by colposcopic biopsy but, if the biopsy is small and superficial, without underlying stroma, then obviously no comment can be made about invasion.

Endocervical curettage

Endocervical curettage (ECC) is widely advocated as part of the routine colposcopic evaluation in the United States, for assessing the state of the epithelium in the cervical canal, but it is not used in the UK to any extent. The material produced by endocervical curettage is scanty, consisting of mucus, blood, fragments of endocervical columnar epithelium and slivers of squamous epithelium. It is unusual for a substantial amount of stroma to be present, so that usually no comment can be made about the presence or absence of invasion. Often all that can be said is that the epithelium is atypical; it may not be possible to assess the degree of CIN in an endocervical curettage specimen. It is important that processing is done carefully and the blocks sectioned at levels. Obviously no attempt at orientation can be made.

LLETZ specimen and cone biopsy

The procedures of large loop excision of the transformation zone (LLETZ) and knife cone biopsy result in generally similar specimens, as does laser excision. The excised tissue should immediately be placed in ample fixative, which is normally formalin. A marker stitch is only of value if the gynaecologist wishes to know the antero-posterior distribution of the lesions; it does not need to be done for the pathologist's benefit. The fixed conization specimen is divided into blocks by parallel sagittal cuts, each 2–3 mm apart. An alternative and widely used method is for the specimen to be opened before fixation and for it to be fixed open, pinned to a piece of cork or wax. This method has the disadvantage that the epithelium lining the canal will inevitably be stretched when the cervix is opened out and fragile abnormal epithelium may be dislodged; for this reason is not recommended

Hysterectomy specimen

If a woman with CIN is treated by hysterectomy, then the cervix is removed from the hysterectomy specimen and handled in the same way as a conization specimen.

LEARNING POINTS

1. Cervical intraepithelial neoplasia is a spectrum of disease, with no clearly-defined diagnostic boundaries within the spectrum or at its lower end, where it merges with physiological changes.
2. There is disagreement as to whether CIN should be classified by division into three or two grades and whether HPV infection should be included with CIN.
3. Increasing grades of severity of CIN show increasing thickness of un-differentiated cells in the epithelium, increasing nuclear abnormalities and an increasing number of mitotic figures. Abnormal mitotic figures are more obvious in the more severe grades but may be seen in CIN 1.
4. The earliest stages of invasion are seen as breaks in the basement membrane with sprouts of squamous cells pushing into the stroma.
5. Slightly more advanced but still very small preclinical carcinomas (microinvasive carcinomas) are assessed by measurement in two dimensions: greatest depth of invasion from the surface and widest lateral spread. These measurements are used to guide management.
6. Punch biopsies should be examined at six levels.
7. Excision specimens (LLETZ and cone biopsies) are serially blocked at 2.0–3.0 mm intervals and entirely embedded. They should not be opened before fixation.

MCQS

7. The following histological features distinguish CIN 3 from CIN 1:
   a. CIN 3 shows greater nuclear pleomorphism than CIN 1
   b. CIN 3 shows greater variation in nuclear size than CIN 1

   c. CIN 3 shows better differentiation than CIN 1
   d. Nuclei at the surface are normal in CIN 1
   e. Nucleoli are more prominent in CIN 1 than in CIN 3

8. The following are histological features of early invasive carcinoma:
   a. Focal lymphocytic infiltrate in the stroma
   b. Anaplasia of the invasive cells
   c. Eosinophilia of the invasive cells
   d. Ulceration of the surface epithelium
   e. Focal condensation of stromal collagen

9. Which of the following statements about CIN are true?
   a. CIN naturally falls into three categories rather than two
   b. The term low-grade squamous intraepithelial lesion includes both CIN 1 and human papillomavirus infection
   c. High-grade squamous intraepithelial lesion is an alternative name for CIN 2
   d. Cervical crypts may be involved by all grades of CIN
   e. Most examples of keratinizing CIN arise from the original squamous epithelium of the ectocervix

4

The colposcope and techniques of colposcopy

M. I. Shafi and J. A. Jordan

HISTORY AND INTRODUCTION

The colposcope is a system that allows both magnification and illumination of the cervix which was first introduced in 1925 by Hans Hinselmann. The primary objective was to diagnose cervical cancer in its earliest stage. Magnification range is usually between 6- and 40-fold. It was not until the 1960s' that colposcopy was taken up by the English speaking countries, which was approximately 20 years after the introduction of the Papanicolaou smear. The colposcopist needs to be fully conversant with both cervical cytology and histopathology to fully appreciate the scientific basis of colposcopic appearances.

BASIC PRINCIPLES

Several types of colposcope are available but all are based on similar principles. The major advances since its introduction have been in the light source, fibreoptic cabling and refinement of the optical systems. The colposcope is usually mounted on a freely movable stand, but can also be fixed to the examination table or wall if desired. The focal length varies between 200 and 300 mm, allowing the colposcopist to conduct an examination comfortably. Attachments to the colposcope may include a monocular teaching arm, a video

Handbook of Colposcopy, edited by David Luesley, Mahmood Shafi and Joe Jordan. Published in 1996 by Chapman & Hall, London. ISBN 0 412 71550 3

camera and a green filter. This green filter allows better definition of vascular architecture by absorbing red light and the blood vessels appear black and prominent.

BASIC EQUIPMENT (FIG. 4.1)

A colposcopy couch is preferable, which allows the patient to be examined in a modified lithotomy position. Either the feet are placed in heel rests or knee rests are used to support the legs. The newer hydraulic couches allow an examination position to be found easily without discomfort to the patient or colposcopist. A chair that can be moved up or down is advantageous for the colposcopist, again allowing the optimal examination position to be found.

Instruments should be readily to hand and placed on a nearby trolley. These should include:

1. bivalve speculum: varying sizes should be available and the largest speculum that can comfortably be inserted should be used – each speculum should be available with a suction tube;
2. cotton wool balls;
3. sponge-holding forceps to hold the cotton wool balls;
4. cotton-tip and jumbo swabs
5. endocervical specula which are useful for examination of the lower endocervical canal;

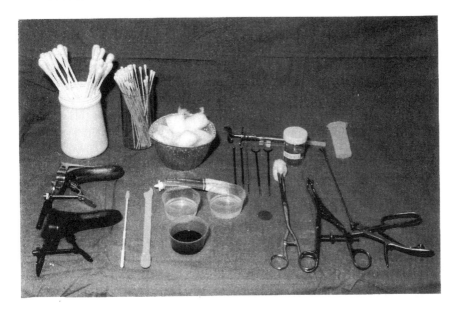

Fig. 4.1 Colposcopy instrument trolley

6. iris hooks, which may be used to manipulate the cervix – a skin hook may be used as a substitute;
7. biopsy forceps: a variety should be available;
8. three small galley pots: these are used to hold normal saline, acetic acid (3% or 5%) and Lugol's iodine;
9. endocervical curette;
10. a variety of loops for use with electrosurgical equipment – these can be used both for biopsy and for therapeutic purposes.

EXAMINATION PROCEDURE

All patients should be examined in warm surroundings and be fully informed about the procedure. Once the patient is comfortable on the examination couch, the cervix is exposed with a bivalve speculum. The cervix and upper vagina are examined at low magnification. If a cervical smear is required, then it should be performed at this stage. Care should be taken to minimize bleeding associated with smear-taking as this may confuse the subsequent assessment. Excess mucus is gently removed from the cervix with a dry or saline-soaked cotton wool ball and the cervix is inspected once again.

Acetic acid (3% or 5%) is gently applied to the cervix and upper vagina with either a cotton wool ball or a jumbo swab, or by using a spray. The acetic acid is left *in situ* for 5–10 seconds and any remaining mucus is relatively easy to remove at this stage. The acetic acid will cause columnar epithelium and abnormal epithelium to appear as white (acetowhite) which is easily distinguishable from the normal, pink squamous epithelium. If the effect of the acetic acid wears off (usually within a minute), reapplication of the acetic acid may be performed. This is important, especially if a permanent record is to be made either using colpophotographs or cervicographs of the abnormality.

Lugol's iodine may be used to outline atypical epithelium as this contains little or no glycogen and therefore will not take up the stain. Normal epithelium, conversely, is glycogen-rich and on application of Lugol's iodine will turn a dark brown colour. Columnar epithelium also contains little or no glycogen and fails to take up the stain. This test is particularly useful for colposcopists who are learning the technique and allows minor degrees of abnormality to be detected which may otherwise have been missed. One area of confusion is that immature metaplasia or congenital transformation zones will also not take up the stain and this may lead to a false-positive result. It is important that these situations are recognized as they are variants of normality.

Some colposcopists will use saline initially prior to application of acetic acid. This technique is particularly useful for the study of angioarchitecture but does require considerable skill in interpretation of the findings.

DOCUMENTATION

This can either be performed using a specially designed colposcopy page or may be stored on computer. Personal preferences will dictate this aspect, which is considered in more detail in Chapter 9.

Terminology

One of the commonest methods of detailing the colposcopy findings is hand-drawn documentation. Diagrams can be added to printed outlines of the cervix, vagina or vulva. For the cervix, it is important to denote the limits of the native squamous epithelium and the transformation zone and to show the new squamocolumnar junction. The position of the anatomical external os should also be noted. Any areas of abnormality are carefully drawn and labelled (Fig. 4.2).

PROBLEMS IN RUNNING A SERVICE

To run an effective cervical cancer prevention programme, we need as a minimum to have cytological screening, diagnostic colposcopy, facilities for histological diagnosis, treatment modalities and follow-up facilities. It is helpful if written guidelines are available in all clinics for the management of patients to cover most eventualities. Contact between the cytologist, colposcopist and histopathologist is essential and an audit programme of the service

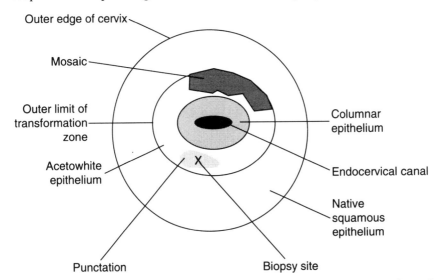

Fig. 4.2 Diagrammatic representation of hand-drawn documentation commonly used to detail colposcopy findings.

should be on-going. There should be good communication with the primary health care team (general practitioners) and with the patients themselves. Literature should be available for distribution to the patients which explains the cervical cancer prevention programme and what will happen to them in the colposcopy clinic. This should be written in plain English and be easily understood.

The clinic layout should be both friendly and efficient. The overall setup will be dependent upon the workload of the department and may vary from a colposcopy room used intermittently to a dedicated facility with colposcopy services available most days.

TRAINING IN COLPOSCOPY

The standard of colposcopy practised in the UK varies from the excellent to the inadequate and this situation is probably similar in most other countries. Other branches of medicine (e.g. ultrasound, psychosexual medicine and family planning) have recognized a similar problem and now offer a diploma or certificate of competence. It is important that women who attend for advice because of an abnormal smear are reassured that they are indeed being seen and advised by a colposcopist who is competent. Similarly, purchasers of colposcopy services need the reassurance that those services are being provided by competent colposcopists.

A system of accreditation in colposcopy will allow national organizations to recommend to purchasers that colposcopy clinics should only be supervised by those who have adequate accreditation or even a diploma of colposcopy. Hospitals would have to ensure that adequately trained staff were employed to provide the colposcopy service. Similarly in clinics staffed by non-specialists, colposcopists need some proof that they are indeed competent to provide the service.

At the end of a training programme a trainee must:

1. be aware of the principles of cervical cytology, histopathology, pathophysiology and basic colposcopy;
2. be able to differentiate low-grade lesions, high-grade lesions and invasive disease of the lower genital tract;
3. be able to decide appropriate management and be thoroughly familiar with all surgical methods of treatment of premalignant and benign disease of the lower genital tract;
4. be able to counsel the woman with abnormal cytology or with a macroscopically abnormal cervix.

To achieve this, it is suggested that a training programme should consist of:

1. attendance at a basic colposcopy course;
2. attendance at 50 colposcopic assessments on women presenting with

abnormal cytology or suspicious lesions in the lower genital tract (direct supervision by a preceptor);
3. 100 colposcopic examinations without direct supervision, each case subsequently being checked with the trainee by the preceptor;
4. the trainee should be deemed competent by the preceptor to advise the woman of treatment options and to perform outpatient treatment;
5. the trainee must be familiar with documentation and audit.

In the future, no one should be allowed to practise colposcopy unsupervised without (1) having been properly trained and (2) having a diploma in colposcopy.

LEARNING POINTS

1. Colposcopy is primarily about magnification and illumination of the cervix.
2. Magnification is usually between 6- and 40-fold.
3. The patient should be warm, relaxed and informed.
4. All basic instruments should be readily available prior to commencing a colposcopic examination.
5. Sequential usage of saline, acetic acid and Lugol's iodine is recommended.
6. The colposcopy findings need to be accurately documented using standard terminology.
7. Training is vital prior to undertaking unsupervised colposcopy.

MCQS

10. With regard to the history of colposcopy:
    a. Colposcopy was introduced by Hans Hinselmann
    b. Colposcopy largely replaced cervical cytology
    c. Commonly used magnifications are up to 100-fold
    d. An understanding of histopathology is useful for practising colposcopists
    e. The green filter has been an important development in the field of colposcopy

11. With regard to equipment in the colposcopy clinic:
    a. A bivalve speculum is ideal to visualize the cervix
    b. Cervical smears should never be taken prior to colposcopy
    c. Nitric acid is an important stain to detect preinvasive changes
    d. An endocervical speculum is useful for examining the lower endocervical canal
    e. Biopsies should only be taken in exceptional circumstances

12. During a colposcopic examination:
    a. The cervix should be fully exposed
    b. For a satisfactory colposcopic assessment, the squamocolumnar junction should be visualized
    c. Normal squamous epithelium fails to stain with Lugol's iodine
    d. Areas of metaplasia are where the squamous epithelium is transforming to columnar epithelium
    e. Only abnormal epithelium turns white with the application of acetic acid

Normal colposcopic appearances

5

J. Murphy

INTRODUCTION

In earlier chapters of this text the anatomy of the cervix was presented in detail. In addition, the various cervical epithelia, their appearance and their relationship to the development of cervical cancer were outlined. The importance of colposcopy in the understanding of the pathophysiology of the cervix was also highlighted, as was a description on colposcopic technique.

Colposcopy, with its unique ability to examine *in situ* the epithelia of the cervix, has allowed the clinician to correlate the appearances of the cervix under direct vision with the histology of these tissues. Colposcopy has been the most significant advance in the management of women with abnormal cervical cytology, and the colposcopic appearances of abnormal cervical epithelia have allowed the clinician to direct the intelligent, and in most cases conservative, treatment of women with cervical intraepithelial neoplasia (CIN). The colposcopic appearances of the abnormal cervix are fascinating, and will be discussed in detail in subsequent chapters.

In common with all aspects of medicine, when considering the cervix, a thorough knowledge of the normal is an essential prerequisite for the study of the abnormal. This chapter examines the colposcopic appearances of normal cervical epithelia: squamous, columnar and metaplastic. The appearances of the normal subepithelial cervical vasculature will also be presented. A knowledge of the appearances of the three types of normal epithelia and

Handbook of Colposcopy, edited by David Luesley, Mahmood Shafi and Joe Jordan. Published in 1996 by Chapman & Hall, London. ISBN 0 412 71550 3

the relationship between them is of first importance in understanding the origins of cervical cancer.

Epithelial types

The cervix has two fundamental types of epithelium: columnar and squamous, both laid down *in utero* and meeting each other in an abrupt fashion at the original squamocolumnar junction (OSCJ) (Fig. 5.1). In ideal, though somewhat theoretical, circumstances the original squamocolumnar junction is situated at the external os. Depending on the size, shape, and configuration of the external os, various proportions of the endocervical canal may be visible.

The position of the OSCJ is variable. It may be completely within the endocervical canal and consequently invisible to the unaided eye, or even to the colposcopist, or it may encroach for a variable degree on to the ectocervix being, in this situation, often described as an ectopy. Using the unaided eye columnar epithelium appears red. This is because the epithelium is very thin and the blood vessels of each columnar villus give a characteristic red colour.

Columnar epithelium

At colposcopy normal epithelium is relatively easy to recognize because of its villus or 'grape-like' appearance. Before the application of acetic acid, and at high colposcopic magnification, it can be observed that each villus has a

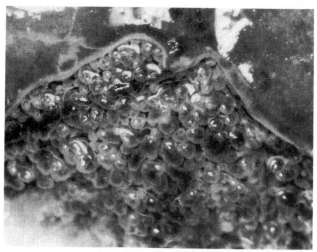

Fig. 5.1 Normal columnar epithelium, showing normal squamous epithelium and the squamocolumnar junction. (Source: reproduced from Murphy, J. (1992) Colposcopic appearances of the normal cervix, in *Integrated Colposcopy*, 1st edn, (ed. M. C. Anderson), Chapman & Hall, London, ch.7, with permission.)

central blood vessel. The blood in the capillaries goes through the single layer of cells and gives the characteristic appearance. Contact bleeding is consequently common, and the epithelial surface can be easily damaged. When acetic acid is applied the villi often appear white and are in general more distinct.

At very high magnification with the scanning or surface electron microscope each columnar villus is covered by a myriad of columnar cells each of which in turn is covered by microvilli (Fig. 5.2).

Squamous epithelium

With colposcopy two types of squamous epithelium may be recognized: original squamous epithelium and transformed or metaplastic squamous epithelium. The original squamous epithelium is formed during fetal development. This epithelium, which covers a variable part of the ectocervix, is similar to the squamous epithelium of the vagina except that stromal papillae are less frequent or even absent. At colposcopy, using ordinary light, it appears smooth, pale and pink in colour and has little apparent vascular pattern. If, however, a green filter is interposed (the technique of Kraatz) in most cases the underlying capillary network becomes apparent (Fig. 5.3).

This network takes the form of tiny, hairpin-like capillaries densely arranged, particularly around the external os. When examined at very high magnification with the scanning electron microscope, squamous epithelium is composed of large flat cells with well developed nuclei arranged in a pavement-like pattern. The surface of these cells is composed of microridges, which

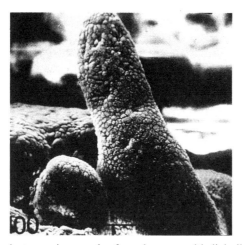

Fig. 5.2 Scanning electron micrograph of a columnar epithelial villus. Each villus is covered by columnar cells. (Source: reproduced from Murphy, J. (1992) Colposcopic appearances of the normal cervix, in *Integrated Colposcopy*, 1st edn, (ed. M. C. Anderson), Chapman & Hall, London, ch.7, with permission.)

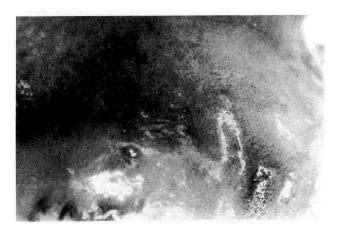

Fig. 5.3   Fine hairpin capillaries. The intercapillary difference varies between 50 and 200 μm. (Source: reproduced from Murphy, J. (1992) Colposcopic appearances of the normal cervix, in *Integrated Colposcopy*, 1st edn, (ed. M. C. Anderson), Chapman & Hall, London, ch.7, with permission.)

interdigitate with those of cells in the lower layers, thus giving this type of epithelium its characteristic strength.

Metaplastic squamous epithelia

To begin to understand the origins of cervical cancer and to use colposcopy intelligently a knowledge of squamous metaplasia is essential. This process has already been extensively discussed in previous chapters. It has been accepted, now for some decades, that columnar epithelium exposed to the vaginal environment tends to change into squamous epithelium by the process of squamous metaplasia. The term 'transformation zone' is used by the colposcopist to describe that part of the cervix which at one stage in its life had been covered by columnar epithelium, but which subsequently changed to squamous epithelium by the process of metaplasia.

Therefore the transformation zone is an area of variable width and configuration lying between the columnar epithelium and the original squamous epithelium. This area contains areas of columnar epithelium and metaplastic squamous epithelium of various stages of maturity. It also contains cervical crypt openings, and at times Nabothian cysts. These cysts occur when a crypt opening becomes covered with metaplastic squamous epithelium and the produced mucous is unable to escape. In the premenopausal woman the transformation zone is usually wholly visible, whereas in the postmenopausal woman, consequent on cervical involution, it can be found in part or totally in the endocervical canal.

The distal limit of the transformation zone is easily defined, usually by a thin line separating the two squamous epithelia of different origin: the native and the metaplastic. This line also represents the position of the original squamocolumnar junction.

RECOGNITION OF MATURE METAPLASIA

Mature metaplastic squamous epithelium can be difficult to distinguish from original squamous epithelium on superficial inspection. However, the presence of crypt openings and branching vessels (to be discussed later) are usually characteristic. Difficulty in interpretation can also arise from the coexistence of less mature metaplastic epithelium.

Immature metaplasia

The early phases of the transformation from columnar to squamous epithelium can be difficult to recognize. The epithelium is acetowhite and can at times be confused with abnormal epithelium. Coppleson and Reid from Sydney, who did so much to make the whole entity of squamous metaplasia understandable, described three colposcopically recognizable stages of squamous metaplasia.

1. The columnar villi lose their translucency and each villus assumes a 'ground glass' appearance.
2. The grape-like configuration disappears as successive villi are fused and the spaces between them are filled in.
3. The villus configuration is lost because of the fusion, and the end result is normal squamous epithelium (Fig. 5.4).

This metaplastic process is, however, patchy, and the process is not all even, or taking place at the same time.

THE VASCULATURE OF THE NORMAL CERVIX

As a knowledge of the vascular pattern seen in epithelial abnormalities of the cervix is so important for their proper interpretation, it stands to reason that the appearances of the vessels in the normal cervix is of significant importance. The part of the cervix covered with columnar epithelium is supplied by branches from the ascending branch of the uterine artery, while that part of the cervix covered by original squamous epithelium is supplied by branches from the cervicovaginal part of the uterine artery and by the vaginal artery. A well developed network of vessels is then formed and the terminal aspects of these vessels can often be seen at colposcopy.

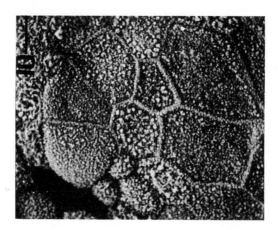

Fig. 5.4 Metaplasia, Stage III. Scanning electron micrograph showing flat, almost mature squamous cells. (Source: reproduced from Murphy, J. (1992) Colposcopic appearances of the normal cervix, in *Integrated Colposcopy*, 1st edn, (ed. M. C. Anderson), Chapman & Hall, London, ch.7, with permission.)

If squamous epithelium is examined in detail and with care, four types of capillaries may be identified. These were first described in detail by two Scandinavian colposcopists, Koller and Kolstad.

Hairpin capillaries

These terminal capillaries are formed by one ascending and one descending branch of fine calibre forming a small loop. Usually only the tip of the loop is visible and the hairpin-like capillaries are recognized as regular and densely arranged small dots (Fig. 5.3).

Network capillaries

Network capillaries are described when the terminal capillaries of the squamous epithelium form a dense, somewhat irregular meshwork of very fine vessels.

Double capillaries

Double capillaries is the term applied to hairpin capillaries that show two or more crests at the top of the loop. These are characteristically found when there is inflammation of the cervical epithelium, particularly with *Trichomonas vaginalis*.

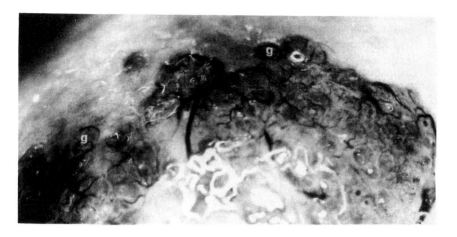

Fig. 5.5 Branching vessels seen in a normal transformation zone. Some are arranged round a gland opening (g). (Source: reproduced from Murphy, J. (1992) Colposcopic appearances of the normal cervix, in *Integrated Colposcopy*, 1st edn, (ed. M. C. Anderson), Chapman & Hall, London, ch.7, with permission.)

Branching vessels

These are larger terminal vessels showing irregular branching patterns (Fig. 5.5). As they decrease in calibre they terminate in a fine-mesh capillary network. They are characteristically seen in the transformation zone and are often prominent in the walls of retention Nabothian cysts. To the uninitiated these might be confused with vascular patterns of invasive cancer but following some experience they can be easily distinguished.

CONCLUSION

It is axiomatic that a thorough knowledge of the normal is essential for understanding the abnormal. In company with other chapters in this text on normal appearances and function, stress must be continually placed on the understanding and recognition of the phenomenon of squamous metaplasia.

LEARNING POINTS

1. Columnar and squamous epithelium are the two basic epithelia laid down *in utero* and join at the original squamocolumnar junction.
2. Columnar epithelium is one cell thick, hence it is easily traumatized.
3. Colposcopy can identify original squamous and metaplastic squamous epithelium.

4. The colposcopic transformation zone represents an area of epithelium that at one stage in its development was columnar epithelium.
5. The transformation zone is variable in width and configuration and contains columnar and squamous metaplastic epithelium of varying maturity.
6. The presence of crypt openings and branching vessels are characteristic of mature squamous metaplastic epithelium.
7. Three stages of metaplasia can be identified colposcopically.

MCQs

13. In colposcopy of the normal cervix:
    a. It is possible to demonstrate three levels of metaplasia
    b. The green filter was introduced by Lugol
    c. The transformation zone can contain columnar epithelium
    d. Metaplasia is smooth, confluent and regular
    e. Double capillaries are suggestive of an inflammatory process

14. At colposcopy, normal columnar epithelium:
    a. Demonstrates a red appearance because of subepithelial haemorrhage
    b. Is characterized by a 'grape-like' appearance
    c. Does not change following the application of 5% acetic acid
    d. Has identifiable villi each with one central capillary
    e. Shows microvilli on the surface of columnar cells

Indications for referral for colposcopy

6

I. D. Duncan

BACKGROUND

Hinselmann introduced the colposcope in 1925 to allow stereoscopic examination of the illuminated cervix under magnification. His main intention was to detect early cervical cancer but he recommended the routine use of the colposcope for every woman undergoing gynaecological examination. The use of the colposcope in this way spread from Germany to Spain and other parts of mainland Europe and from there to South America. The English-speaking world, including the UK, does not use colposcopy for primary screening for cervical premalignancy. Cervical cytology is routinely used in this respect and the colposcope is reserved for those women in whom a diagnosis of cervical intraepithelial neoplasia (CIN) is suspected. Neither cytology nor colposcopy is 100% sensitive or specific. False negatives and false positives occur with both methods. They are, however, complementary and the accuracy of using both methods in combination is greater than using either method in isolation. It is easier and quicker, however, to gain expertise in taking a smear than in carrying out colposcopy and the cytological impression, unlike the colposcopic one, does not require the physical presence of the woman herself. For socioeconomic reasons, if for no other, it is highly unlikely that primary screening with colposcopy will become established as routine practice in the UK. It is important, therefore, that the indications for colposcopy are clearly set out.

Handbook of Colposcopy, edited by David Luesley, Mahmood Shafi and Joe Jordan. Published in 1996 by Chapman & Hall, London. ISBN 0 412 71550 3

GUIDELINES FOR REFERRAL

In 1981 the Working Party set up by the Royal College of Obstetricians and Gynaecologists recommended that no woman should be treated for CIN without first undergoing colposcopy. This recommendation remains sacrosanct. Priority should be given to the detection of CIN 3 over CIN 1 since the risk of CIN 3 progressing through microinvasion to frank invasive cancer of the cervix is greater than for CIN 1, which is more likely to regress to normality than CIN 3. The correlation between cytology and histology is not 100% but it does approach this figure at the extremes, i.e. a woman with a negative smear is unlikely to have CIN and a woman with severe dyskaryosis is likely to have high-grade CIN. In 1992 guidelines were published for clinical practice and programme management for use in the NHS cervical screening programme. These guidelines contain the recommendation that women with a smear showing moderate or severe dyskaryosis should be referred for colposcopy straight away.

Low-grade cervical cytology does not necessarily correlate with low-grade histological abnormality. Various centres have demonstrated the existence of CIN 2 or 3 on colposcopically directed biopsy in women whose worst cytological abnormality is mild dyskaryosis. This is not because of faulty technique in either taking, preparing or reading the smear but appears to be due to the fact that the high-grade lesion present in a woman with only mild dyskaryosis is very much smaller than when severe dyskaryosis is seen on the smear. Thus a high-grade lesion must have a critical surface area before it is sufficiently represented on the smear and the inaccuracy of low-grade cytology is a constant phenomenon. The national guidelines recognize this and recommend that women with a borderline or mildly dyskaryotic smear should have it repeated 6 months later and consideration only given to colposcopic referral if the repeat smear is not normal.

OTHER REFERRAL SITUATIONS

Although the basis for colposcopic referral is abnormal cytology there are other situations in which colposcopy may be useful. In some young women the degree of cervical eversion and the fragility of the exposed columnar epithelium is such that the cervix bleeds readily when a smear is taken and the red blood cells may be sufficient to obscure the cervical cells so that the smear is reported as unsatisfactory (Chapter 2). If the smears are repeatedly unsatisfactory the colposcopist may be called upon to examine the cervix and pronounce it normal or not.

In the UK, cervical screening is predominantly carried out in general practice and with increasing frequency by the practice nurse, who is less and less likely to encounter cervical cancer. Benign conditions, e.g. condylomata acuminata, can give rise to the suspicion of cancer and even if the cytology is negative the exceptional case should be referred for colposcopic examination.

PRIMARY SCREENING COLPOSCOPY

Primary screening with colposcopy is sometimes used in genito-urinary medicine clinics. In the UK the population attending these clinics tends to be younger women with a higher prevalence of Human papillomavirus infection and CIN, especially low-grade, than in the general population. Concomitant sexually transmitted inflammatory conditions of the cervix such as infection with *Trichomonas vaginalis* or *Chlamydia trachomatis* may again make cytology less reliable and the addition of colposcopy a useful adjunct.

COLPOSCOPY OF OTHER STRUCTURES

Although primarily designed for examination of the cervix the colposcope can be used to look at other structures such as the vulva or penis. The vascular pattern is less apparent in these structures since the skin is thicker than the cervical epithelium. Nuclear-rich tissues will still temporarily turn white after the application of acetic acid, although the process is slower than in the cervix. Vulvar intraepithelial neoplasia (VIN) and penile intraepithelial neoplasia (PIN) are much less common than CIN. VIN is usually symptomatic, the commonest symptom being pruritus or soreness. The lesions may be seen with the naked eye. They are commonly multifocal and may be red or brown, or white if there is increased keratinization present. Penile lesions may be unsuspected but can be located on the shaft of the penis of the male partners of women with CIN, especially those with persistent or recurrent CIN. A hand lens as used by the dermatologist can be a simple substitute for the colposcope.

The carbon dioxide laser is still commonly used to treat these lesions despite the fact that recurrence is likely and of course the colposcope is usually an integral part of such a laser system.

CONCLUSION

Squamous cervical cancer is largely preventable. Well established cytology programmes have been rewarded by a fall in incidence of the condition but false negatives still occur. In addition, large numbers of women with minor lesions, the vast majority of which are not precancerous, are caught in the net and end up being investigated and often treated. Trials are under way checking the Human papillomavirus (HPV) status of women when the smear is taken.

HPV 16 and 18 are the more common of the so called high-risk oncogenic group and are associated with high-grade intraepithelial neoplasia and cancer while HPV 6 and 11 are characteristic of the low-risk group and predominate in low-grade lesions. Again correlation between histology and HPV status is not 100%. A few low-grade lesions will contain high-risk virus and a few high-grade lesions will contain low-risk virus. In the future it is possible that HPV status may be used to refine referral for colposcopy.

The national guidelines also contain recommendations for the follow-up of women who have undergone treatment for CIN. Cytology is essential in these women. Colposcopy has been shown to aid in the early detection of persistent lesions and may be used at the 6-month follow-up visit. If, however, that examination, which is optional, is negative it need not be repeated. Women in the UK find colposcopy at best distasteful and at worst a frightening, humiliating procedure. Referral for colposcopy must therefore be a careful balance between the benefits likely to accrue to the women and the psychological trauma of an unnecessary intrusive examination.

LEARNING POINTS

1. Moderate and severe dyskaryosis are indications for referral for colposcopy.
2. Any suspicious-looking cervical lesion is an indication for referral regardless of the cytology report.
3. Mild dyskaryosis and borderline changes should prompt a repeat smear 6 months after the index smear. If any abnormality persists, referral is recommended. These guidelines are based upon a common consensus and not on the evidence of clinical trials.
4. Colposcopy is not generally regarded as a screening process.
5. Between 20% and 40% of women who have low-grade smear reports (mild dyskaryosis and borderline nuclear abnormalities) will have CIN 2 or CIN 3 on biopsy. These lesions tend to be smaller than those presenting with high-grade cytological abnormalities.
6. The colposcope is primarily designed for examination of the cervix. Examination of other areas of the female lower genital tract and the penis may be enhanced by using the colposcope.

MCQS

15. The following are indications for colposcopy in the UK:
    a. A single mildly dyskaryotic smear
    b. A single moderately dyskaryotic smear
    c. A single severely dyskaryotic smear

d. A cervical polyp
e. A routine follow-up visit 18 months after treatment for CIN 3

16. Which of the following statements about cervical smears are true?
   a. There is a high correlation between negative cytology and negative histology
   b. There is a poor correlation between low-grade cytology and low-grade histology
   c. There is a high correlation between high-grade cytology and high-grade histology
   d. HPV 16 is a high-risk oncogenic virus
   e. HPV 6 is a high-risk oncogenic virus

17. Colposcopy:
   a. Was first developed in Germany
   b. Is used as a screening tool in some genito-urinary medicine clinics in the UK
   c. Is usually performed at a magnification of × 40
   d. Is only used to examine female anatomy
   e. Is essential in the diagnosis of VIN

Colposcopy of the atypical transformation zone

J. Cordiner

INTRODUCTION

The atypical transformation zone is that area of the cervix whose limits define cervical intraepithelial neoplasia. A comprehensive understanding of the normal anatomy, the physiology and colposcopy is necessary to interpret abnormal findings. Unfortunately there is no single feature capable of defining a distinct histological abnormality.

It is important that the cervix be viewed prior to the application of acetic acid as many of the features suggestive of cervical intraepithelial neoplasia are present when viewed microscopically, especially when accentuated by gently cleansing the area with saline and visualizing with a green filter *in situ*. However, the majority of colposcopy clinics in the UK will use the acetic acid technique to delineate the abnormal transformation zone.

THE ATYPICAL TRANSFORMATION ZONE

Acetowhite epithelium

This is a focal abnormal colposcopic appearance after the application of acetic acid (Plate 1). It is a transient phenomenon associated with increased nuclear density. It is the most commonly found of all abnormal features associated with the abnormal transformation zone but is not diagnostic of CIN. It may

Handbook of Colposcopy, edited by David Luesley, Mahmood Shafi and Joe Jordan. Published in 1996 by Chapman & Hall, London. ISBN 0 412 71550 3

be found in association with Human papillomavirus (HPV) infection, immature squamous metaplasia, congenital transformation zone and regenerating epithelium.

In general, the more intense the change, the more extreme the degree of histological abnormality. The ectocervical edge may be clear and well defined or fuzzy, the latter often associated with HPV infection.

Vascular pattern

The viewed pattern and calibre of the subepithelial capillaries frequently give a striking colposcopic appearance. There are three clearly identifiable types.

Mosaic

This is a focal abnormal colposcopic appearance in which the vascular patterns show fields of mosaic within the transformation zone (Plate 2). The capillaries appear parallel to the surface, giving the characteristic crazy paving pattern. The calibre of the capillaries may vary as may the surface area enclosed. The wider the calibre and the greater the surface area enclosed, the more likely a greater degree of abnormality.

Punctation

The stromal capillaries produce a stippled or punctate appearance within the epithelium (Plate 3). The degree of punctation may be fine with evenly spaced loop capillaries of narrow calibre with minimal intercapillary distance. In a more marked change, the course and calibre of the capillaries is altered, with coarse-calibre vessels often called and resembling corkscrews. In general the more severe the change the greater the degree of histological abnormality. In many inflammatory states the subepithelial capillaries open up and again produce a stippled effect.

This should not be confused with punctation associated with an abnormal transformation zone as the punctation in inflammatory change is diffuse and extends on to the original squamous epithelium in the vagina and fornices.

Atypical vessels

These vessels are frequently arranged in a haphazard way (Plate 4). New vessels are formed and often demonstrate gross variation in calibre and branching. At the extreme, the appearances of atypical vessels are suggestive that early invasion of the stroma may have taken place. The vessels themselves are different from vascular patterns seen in the normal transformation zone. Fine terminal branching is uncommon with atypical vessels.

If acetic acid is used, the vascular appearance of the transformation zone may be obliterated by dense acetowhite epithelium. The pattern may not be obvious until the effect of the acetic acid wears off.

GRADING OF COLPOSCOPIC FINDINGS

There is no one feature of the abnormal transformation zone which is diagnostic. It has therefore been customary to grade the findings.

Grade I

The epithelium is flat and white with fine-calibre, regular blood vessels and a small intercapillary distance.

Grade II

The epithelium remains flat but is whiter after the application of acetic acid. The vessels are usually regular but perhaps of a larger diameter, with increased intercapillary distance.

Grade III

The epithelium is intensely acetowhite; the blood vessels are dilated and irregular with frequently a variable intercapillary distance. There may be atypical vessels. The surface in early invasive cancer may be uneven, papillary or exophytic. The variations of the surface contour and the vessels are often coincident but one may exist without the other. The appearance of atypical vessels and a grossly irregular surface contour is highly suggestive of invasive carcinoma.

LEUKOPLAKIA

This is a focal appearance in which there is hyperkeratosis or parakeratosis. It appears on colposcopy as an elevated, roughened, white area prior to the application of acetic acid. Some of the keratin may be washed away using a saline-soaked swab, thereby leaving a glistening whitened appearance. It may be patchy or cover large areas of the cervix and may extend outside the transformation zone on to the vagina. Its significance is that it may obscure the visualization of the surface and vascular architecture of the transformation zone. Biopsy is required.

VAGINAL EXTENSION OF CIN

In the majority of cases encountered in women of reproductive years, it will be possible to visualize the whole transformation zone on the cervix. In a small number of cases (about 5%) there may be vaginal extension of the transformation zone on to the vaginal vault. This may occur for two reasons.

Vaginal extension of intraepithelial disease

There has been genuine metaplastic/dysplastic change taking place on the extended transformation zone. The appearances colposcopically will be similar to those on the cervix with acetowhite epithelium and altered angioarchitecture. The limits are often well defined after application of Lugol's iodine, as the area does not take up the iodine stain.

Congenital transformation zone

This concept is often confusing to both experienced and inexperienced colposcopists. Under normal circumstances, columnar epithelium undergoing the physiological change of metaplasia reaches full maturation, the resulting squamous epithelium being indistinguishable from normal. In a small but often confusing number of patients, the metaplastic change results in an acetowhite epithelium which is non-glycogenated. The majority of this change is on the cervix, but it may extend on to the vaginal vault. This is the congenital transformation zone. On visualization of this after the application of acetic acid, it is often slow to become white and slow to return to normal. There is often an extremely fine mosaic of thin-calibre vessels on its surface. The epithelium is poorly or non-glycogenated. The appearances are often confusing and frequently biopsy is required to confirm the classic histological features of the congenital transformation zone. Its potential for malignancy is low and treatment is not required.

ENDOCERVICAL EXTENSION OF TRANSFORMATION ZONE

While in cases of CIN the ectocervical limits of a lesion are often clear and well demarcated, the endocervical limits are frequently less well defined. In many woman in late reproductive life or postmenopausal women the transformation zone will extend to beyond the visual limits of the colposcope. An endocervical speculum may be helpful to define the upper limit but as the incident light from the colposcope is not at right angles to the lesion, the appearances can occasionally be confusing. Excision biopsy should be undertaken should there be any doubt about the upper limit of the transformation zone.

HPV APPEARANCES AND COLPOSCOPY

There is increasing evidence of the strong association between Human papillomavirus and the development of cervical precancer and cancer.

EDUCATION CENTRE LIBRARY
FURNESS GENERAL HOSPITAL
BARROW-IN-FURNESS

Colposcopic evidence of HPV infection may vary from clearly defined exophytic warts through non-condylomatous warts and indeed to virtually normal colposcopic appearances.

Condyloma acuminata

The classical lesions of wart virus infection may be visible to the naked eye. They have multiple papillary projections, each with its own looped capillary. An important feature is that such lesions are not confined to the transformation zone and they extend out on to the vagina and to the lower genital tract. On colposcopy each individual wart has a frond-like surface and central capillary. This is often better visualized prior to the application of acetic acid. With the application of acetic acid there is intense blanching of the surface; this frequently persists for some time. Occasionally the surface of the wart has an appearance likened to human brain (encephaloid appearance) in which the surface is heaped up and has a whorled appearance. As such lesions are frequently associated with CIN, biopsy is often required.

Flat warts (non-condylomatous wart virus infection)

To document the classical appearance of subclinical papillomavirus infections is difficult. The appearances are often subtle and indistinct. The surface of the epithelium is often shiny and off-white. The margins of the lesion are often irregular and pointed and have a feathery appearance. There may indeed be satellite lesions outside the transformation zone. There may be fine punctation with a fine mosaic pattern of the underlying vessels. Several authors have attempted to score appearances to simplify the classification but although they may be helpful in the training of the colposcopist, biopsy of the lesion is often the only way to determine whether underlying CIN is present.

UNSATISFACTORY COLPOSCOPY

It is the function of colposcopy and the colposcopist to be able to define the outer and inner limits of the transformation zone, to make an interpretation of these findings, to enable appropriate biopsy and treatment to be undertaken. Colposcopy is deemed to be unsatisfactory when it is not possible to do this. It may be a simple fact that visualization of the cervix is poor or that the transformation zone extends into the endocervical canal and outside the visual range. In certain circumstances, coexisting lesions may cause some confusion.

Inflammatory changes

A wide range of causes exist for this. Common organisms such as *Candida albicans*, *Trichomonas vaginalis* and *Neisseria gonorrhoeae* may produce a severe vascular response. On colposcopy the appearances are compatible with hyperaemia of the vascular capillary bed. The terminal capillaries become dilated and often looped in an accentuated normal response. This produces an intense punctation but, in contradistinction to the atypical transformation zone, the vessels are close together and will usually extend on to the vaginal epithelium.

Atrophic epithelium

Colposcopy of oestrogen deficient epithelium is often confusing. The epithelium becomes pale, white and thin. The full subepithelial network of capillaries is often visualized through the thinned epithelium and subepithelial haemorrhage is common.

True erosion

This is an area of denuded epithelium, usually caused by trauma. On colposcopy the exposed area is red, as the terminal vessels are visualized. The epithelium is lifted off the crater base and can be easily identified.

SUMMARY

It is important that the colposcopist detects the abnormal colposcopic appearances of premalignant and early malignant disease. As has been emphasized, no one appearance is classical and appearances can often be confusing. Biopsy of any areas of doubt is the only method to determine whether treatment is required or not.

LEARNING POINTS

1. No one colposcopic feature is diagnostic of cervical intraepithelial neoplasia.
2. The vascular pattern of the subendothelial capillary network should be first assessed after the application of normal saline and using a green filter.
3. In general, the coarser the vascular pattern and more intense the whiteness after the application of acetic acid, the worse the degree of CIN.
4. Human papillomavirus and immature metaplasia may also result in acetowhite changes.
5. Atypical vessels and an irregular surface contour are suggestive of underlying invasion.
6. Leukoplakia can mask underlying CIN.

7. Acetowhite epithelium extending on to the vagina may represent either true dysplastic extension (VaIN) or a congenital transformation zone.
8. The colposcopic features of HPV infection are subtle and can be confused with mild dysplastic change. Extension of atypicality beyond the transformation zone is, however, suggestive of HPV.
9. Inflammatory processes can cause marked changes in the subepithelial capillary network. These changes also extend beyond the transformation zone.

MCQs

18. The transformation zone (TZ):
    a. Is delineated as the area below the SCJ
    b. That shows acetowhitening is pathognomonic of CIN
    c. That shows a mosaic pattern has low-grade CIN
    d. That shows diffuse punctation extending on to the original squamous epithelium suggests an inflammatory process
    e. Fine terminal vessel branching is not usually associated with atypical vessels

19. HPV infection:
    a. Is always clearly defined colposcopically
    b. Is not confined to the transformation zone
    c. Can have an encephaloid appearance
    d. Has clearly defined margins when seen colposcopically
    e. Can usefully be categorized by using scoring systems

20. Inflammatory changes:
    a. Are always associated with bacterial infection
    b. Can be caused by *Candida albicans*
    c. Are present in schistosomal infection
    d. May be similar to atrophic changes on colposcopy
    e. On colposcopy, the appearances are compatible with hyperaemia of the vascular bed

Abnormal colposcopy (early invasion, glandular lesions)

C. W. E. Redman

INTRODUCTION

This chapter focuses on the colposcopic assessment of early invasive and glandular cervical lesions. The term 'glandular lesions' can embrace a histopathological spectrum of endocervical abnormality from mild atypia, through the more severe adenocarcinoma-*in-situ* (AIS) to frank invasive adenocarcinoma, but only AIS and adenocarcinoma will be considered here. Early invasion is synonymous with preclinical cancer of FIGO stage Ia1 (early stromal invasion) and stage Ia2 (microinvasion). Histopathological aspects and management are described elsewhere.

Colposcopy is necessary for the optimal management of women with abnormal cervical cytology or suspicious clinical features but the actual colposcopic assessment *per se* consists only partly of the necessary information. Other important clinical features include the history, examination findings and certain investigations. This chapter aims to describe the detection and assessment of early invasive and glandular lesions more fully than simply detailing specifically what might be seen looking down a colposcope. There are no colposcopic features diagnostic of a glandular lesion. The colposcope merely serves to increase suspicion of such a lesion. Diagnosis is a histological one.

Handbook of Colposcopy, edited by David Luesley, Mahmood Shafi and Joe Jordan. Published in 1996 by Chapman & Hall, London. ISBN 0 412 71550 3

THE IMPORTANCE OF EARLY INVASIVE AND GLANDULAR LESIONS

These lesions histopathologically occupy a grey area between preinvasive and frankly invasive cancer and this is reflected in attitudes and recommendations about treatment. Appropriate treatment depends on accurate diagnosis and it is now clear that prior to the advent of loop diathermy excision these lesions were significantly underdiagnosed and undertreated even by expert colposcopists. The clinical challenge posed by these lesions has diminished with the increasing use of loop diathermy.

INDEX OF SUSPICION

Such severe lesions are at one end of the spectrum of disease that is seen in a colposcopy clinic and are uncommon. There is therefore a danger that these cases can easily be overlooked against a background of accompanying minor pathology. Such lesions are too uncommon to be specifically targeted by the screening programme which is aimed instead at detecting and treating high-grade disease, principally CIN 3. There are, however, certain features other than cytology that should alert the clinician to the possibility of invasive disease.

Symptoms

Postcoital, intermenstrual and of course postmenopausal bleeding are all symptoms that have a sinister significance till proven otherwise. In the case of genuine postcoital bleeding there is an argument for assessment to routinely include cervical loop diathermy excision.

Past history

A previous history of treatment for a high-grade cervical lesion, particularly if the lesion was incompletely excised or if the treatment was ablative, should lower the threshold of suspicion. In any event the proven limitations of colposcopy following treatment make histological assessment important should problems arise.

Examination findings

In addition to the clinical appearance of the cervix bimanual examination may raise the possibility of frank invasion because the cervix feels either hard and irregular or abnormal in shape or size. However, early invasive lesions will be subclinical.

COLPOSCOPIC FEATURES SUGGESTING INVASION

Invasive lesions may be clinically apparent, presenting with ulceration or obvious topographical hypertrophy. However not all lesions will be clinically apparent when a patient is first seen.

Classically a number of colposcopic features are considered to be suggestive of invasion. These features simply represent one end of a spectrum of the colposcopic grading of atypical lesions and may not all be evident in any given case. Prior to the application of acetic acid invasion may be obvious from the bizarre appearance of the cervix, if the surface is grossly distorted or ulcerated, or from the presence of abnormal vessels. By and large the application of acetic acid accentuates the features that indicate microinvasive disease (Plates 5, 6).

Abnormal vessels

Markedly atypical and prominent vessels are said to be the hallmark and can have a number of appearances:

1. coarse irregular vessels with a variety of forms (e.g. 'corkscrew' and 'comma') (Plates 7, 8);
2. coarse punctation;
3. 'atypical vessels' – those seen with irregular calibre and usually irregular branching with a wide intercapillary distance.

These features are often very prominent if the lesion is hypertrophic. When there is ulceration they are less obvious.

Irregular surface

The presence of an uneven or raised surface must suggest the possibility of invasion. Invasive cancer is characterized by an irregular and exophytic growth pattern.

Large, complex lesion

There is a positive correlation between lesion size and the histological severity. The larger the lesion the more likely it is to be high-grade. Complex patterns represent a combination of acetowhite, mosaic and punctation.

Severe changes with canal involvement

Any of these features would suggest that an adequate biopsy, such as loop diathermy excision or formal knife cone biopsy, is indicated.

PROBLEMS IN THE RECOGNITION OF EARLY INVASION

Colposcopy may suggest early invasion when it is not there (false positive) or, more worryingly, miss it when it is there (false negative). Overall, colposcopy has not been shown to be particularly accurate, especially in the context of microinvasive disease. It should be regarded as a technique for guiding biopsy and treatment by indicating the likely underlying histological diagnosis in conjunction with other data items, such as cytology, smoking and past history.

False positives are not a major problem. They may result in some unnecessary intervention but most of these lesions will nonetheless be high-grade CIN if not invasive lesions and therefore would require treatment in any event. When invasion is suspected, histological confirmation prior to more extensive therapy is mandatory and at this stage the error will be detected. Such errors should be unusual, although the number will depend on the individual's threshold for making such decisions. False positives are more likely in pregnancy, as the vascular pattern tends to be more exaggerated.

False negatives are, on the other hand, an important problem because early invasive lesions will either not be treated appropriately or even not treated at all. The advent of loop diathermy excision has resulted in a sudden increase in the incidence of early invasion, even in centres of excellence, which means that early invasive lesions were previously missed and inappropriately managed.

A number of factors make false negatives more common.

Previous treatment

The scarring and deformation of the cervical transformation zone resulting from previous treatment, particularly if ablative, makes colposcopy unreliable.

Endocervical lesions

Colposcopy cannot assess any lesion that is hidden from view, for instance when the SCJ is within the endocervical canal.

Leukoplakia

Leukoplakia is not itself indicative of malignancy but as it may mask an underlying lesion it should be biopsied.

Pregnancy

There is a natural tendency to avoid any intervention in pregnancy and therefore a reluctance to perform colposcopy. Colposcopy can be more technically demanding and its findings difficult to interpret.

CAN GLANDULAR LESIONS BE RECOGNIZED?

Frankly invasive adenocarcinoma or adenosquamous carcinoma of the cervix will have similar appearances to squamous lesions. However, there are major limitations in the colposcopic assessment of suspected glandular lesions, as severe preinvasive glandular lesions such as AIS have no typical colposcopic appearance. The only clue may be increased fragility or coexistent CIN.

Frankly invasive glandular lesions will present in a similar manner to the commoner squamous cancers. AIS either presents as an abnormal glandular smear or is found coincidentally in the course of the management of squamous dyskaryosis. Abnormal glandular smears have a variety of forms ranging from 'endometrial' cells being found in cervical smears in inappropriate phases of the menstrual cycle through more marked glandular dyskaryosis to the positive detection of adenocarcinoma cells. The possibility of AIS or worse has to be considered throughout the spectrum of these cytological reports although most 'glandular' smears are only mild and not associated with any significant pathology.

COLPOSCOPIC ASSESSMENT WHEN SMEARS HAVE MILD GLANDULAR ABNORMALITIES

There is an argument that loop diathermy is indicated in the assessment of all women having smears showing a glandular abnormality, as this is the only way to satisfactorily assess the endocervical canal. This would be an overreaction, as most mildly glandular smears need not reflect underlying dysplasia. Currently assessment includes:

1. consideration of whether there may be endometrial pathology and performing an endometrial sample if indicated;
2. performing an endocervical Cytobrush examination – if this provides further evidence of cytological atypia then loop diathermy excision should be performed.

ASSESSMENT WHEN INVASION OR SEVERE GLANDULAR LESIONS ARE SUSPECTED COLPOSCOPICALLY

Histological confirmation

In these circumstances histological confirmation is mandatory. There are, however, a number of considerations.

1. **The biopsy must be sufficient to allow adequate pathological assessment.** Histology can be inadequate in two ways. Firstly, not enough material may be provided. In this respect a punch biopsy is totally inadequate. Few

colposcopists would knowingly use a punch biopsy to confirm a colpo-scopic diagnosis of microinvasion but early invasive lesions are often not suspected colposcopically. It follows that punch biopsies are of dubious value. Secondly, the diagnosis of microinvasion or AIS can only be safely made when the entire lesion has been removed, which may be better assessed after a knife cone biopsy as opposed to a loop diathermy, as the margins of excision are clearer.

2. **Frank invasion may be suspected.** It is pointless performing a large cone biopsy with its attendant dangers to confirm a diagnosis that is clinically obvious. In these circumstance a piece of cervix can be removed either digitally or using a loop.

Staging

Whenever an early invasive lesion is suspected a bimanual pelvic examination should be performed to exclude the possibility of local spread should the definitive histology be Stage Ib. Other investigations such as chest X-ray and intravenous urogram can be deferred until histology is to hand.

LEARNING POINTS

1. Markedly abnormal vessels are highly suggestive of early invasive disease.
2. Despite there being well described colposcopic features, microinvasive lesions are frequently underdiagnosed.
3. If microinvasion is suspected adequate histological confirmation is mandatory.
4. Glandular lesions have no reliable colposcopic features.

MCQS

21. With regard to subclinical invasive lesions of the cervix:
     a. The majority will be accurately diagnosed by colposcopy
     b. If suspected, formal knife cone biopsy is mandatory
     c. Leukoplakia is highly predictive that such lesions are present
     d. Abnormal vessels are highly suggestive
     e. Pregnancy changes may mask the usual colposcopic features

22. The following statements are true:
     a. When glandular lesions are suspected excisional biopsy must be performed
     b. When frank invasion is apparent diagnostic cone biopsy is mandatory

c. Coarse punctation is a cardinal colposcopic feature of adenocarcinoma-*in-situ*
d. Early invasive lesions are likely to have wide intercapillary distances
e. Acetic acid application can mask abnormal vascular patterns

9 | Recording the information

D. M. Luesley and M. I. Shafi

BACKGROUND

Colposcopic assessments, just like any other form of medical assessment, require documentation. This is important for clinical use (future visits), audit and research. Increasingly, established clinics have now developed a standard format for note-taking and image-recording. These usually take the form of a structured or semistructured form for recording important aspects of the history and relevant clinical findings. It must be stressed that colposcopy clinics are specialized clinics for the assessment and management of women with abnormal cervical smears or clinically suspicious cervices. Other clinical problems may also be present, such as menorrhagia or pelvic pain; ideally, these should not be dealt with within the context of the colposcopy clinic. It follows that, unless there are good clinical reasons, bimanual examinations are not indicated as part of a routine colposcopic assessment.

Using a structured format allows important items of data to be captured on all patients and also allows transfer of such information to electronic media for storage and analysis. Developing the use of computers further allows repetitive tasks such as letter writing and appointment scheduling to be done automatically and also allows fail-safe mechanisms to be built into the system (such as routinely flagging missing results, highlighting invasive histology, etc.). Electronic technology also allows for networking, thus bringing together the laboratories, clinic and primary care agencies such as the FHSA who operate the recall system.

Handbook of Colposcopy, edited by David Luesley, Mahmood Shafi and Joe Jordan. Published in 1996 by Chapman & Hall, London. ISBN 0 412 71550 3

BASIC MINIMUM DATASET

Whatever system is employed, from the most basic to the most advanced, it is important to adopt a basic minimum dataset. Each clinic may well decide upon its own priorities. An example of a semistructured dataset that has been in use in our clinic for many years is seen in Figs 9.1 and 9.2.

In general terms the following should be included.

Basic patient information

1. Name (last and first)
2. Date of birth
3. Identification number (unique identifier)
4. Address (including postcode)
5. Obstetric history
6. Contraception
7. Smoking (current and previous)
8. LMP
9. Pregnant, non-pregnant or menopausal
10. Relevant past medical or surgical history (especially cervical surgery)
11. Previous sexually transmitted diseases (especially HPV)
12. GP name and address
13. Source of referral

Note that this list does not contain any information relating to age at first coitus, number of partners, etc. It is the authors' opinion that this does not contribute to patient care in any way, is unlikely to shed any further light on the epidemiology of cervical cancer and precancer (unless as part of a specifically designed epidemiological study), is unnecessarily intrusive and only adds weight to the stigma that many women feel is attached to having an abnormal smear.

Specific disease information

1. Date of most recent cervical smear
2. Grade of most recent smear
3. Date of last normal smear
4. Date and grade of worst smear
5. Previous treatment or biopsies (with dates)
6. Any associated symptoms (PCB, PMB, etc.)

SPECIFIC VISIT INFORMATION

1. Smear taken? if yes, result
2. Biopsy taken? if yes, type and result

Attach patient ID label

Total number of pregnancies	
Total number of live births	

Pregnant now   Yes [ ]   No [ ]   EDD

Post-menopausal   Yes [ ]   No [ ]   LMP

Current contraception
     None   [ ]
     COC   [ ]
     POP   [ ]
     Depot   [ ]
     IUCD   [ ]
     Sheath   [ ]
     Diaphragm   [ ]
     Female Sterilization   [ ]
     Male Sterilization   [ ]
     Other...................................

Previous COC use   Yes [ ]   No [ ]

Previous Infections
     HPV   [ ]
     HSV   [ ]
     Other STD   [ ]

Smoking Status
     Non-smoker   [ ]
     Previous smoker   [ ]
     Current smoker   [ ]...............Per Day
     Partner smokes   [ ]

Using immunosuppressants   Yes [ ]   No [ ]

Date of most recent smear   Result

Date of worst smear   Result

Previous cervical biopsy   Yes [ ]   No [ ]

Previous default from clinic   Yes [ ]   No [ ]

Fig. 9.1 An example of a data recording sheet for new attenders in a colposcopy clinic.

REFERRAL SOURCE		SALUTATION:

Visit number

Prior treatment   Y   N   SPECIFY:

Last cytology report   Date

Last histology report   Date

Type   LMP

Previous pregnancies

COLPOSCOPIST: .... Visit date:

Smear repeated..........   Normal......   WARTS
Smear NOT repeated..   CIN [   ]......   None.........
SCJ seen.....................   ESI............   Suspect.....
SCJ NOT seen.............   Uncertain...   Macro........
  Not Done...   Vaginal......

Stenosed Os
Y   N

CYTOLOGY RESULT

HISTOLOGY RESULT

PROCEDURE AT THIS VISIT   PLANNED ACTION   DEFAULTER

None.........................   Loop excision [LA]......   Send again
Laser........................   Loop excision [GA].....   Discharge
Punch biopsy.............   Cone biopsy...............
Loop excision.............   Other biopsy...............   DISPOSAL
Cone biopsy..............   Hysterectomy..............   G.P
Other biopsy..............   Wertheims..................   Other clinic
Eletrodiathermy..........   Staging.......................   Other Hospital
Hysterectomy.............   Colposcopy F.U. ....
Wertheims.................   Cytology F.U. ....   Letter

Other action/Comments:

Additional history [continued overleaf if neccessary]

Signature:......................

Fig. 9.2 An example of a data sheet for recording details of attendance at a colposcopy clinic.

3. Colposcopy
   a. SCJ seen?
   b. Lesion seen?
   c. Site and size of lesion
   d. Colposcopic opinion
   e. HPV present?
   f. Distorted cervical anatomy (i.e. stenosis)?
   g. Normal vagina?
   h. Normal vulva?
4. Treatment – type? Complications?
5. Information given to patient

FOLLOW-UP INFORMATION

1. Needs treatment: what, where (inpatient or outpatient), when?
2. Needs colposcopy (with or without cytology): where and when?
3. Cytology only: where and when?

It will have become apparent that some of this information does not readily lend itself to simple recording or yes/no-type answers. This is particularly the case for recording the colposcopic image. Why bother to record it at all?

REASONS FOR RECORDING THE COLPOSCOPIC IMAGE

The main reason is for comparison at future visits, especially when the decision is to observe rather than treat. A second reason is for audit purposes. This is particularly the case when one is on the learning curve and trying to match colposcopic expertise with histological outcome. Both of these reasons alone are sufficient to demand some form of recording. Again there is a wide variation in recording techniques and accuracy.

Image recording techniques

The most widely used and least accurate is a simple hand drawing. These are usually not to scale, only record the presence or absence of a lesion and may also specify whether or not the whole transformation zone was visualized. A fairly good example of a hand-drawn recording of a colposcopic assessment is detailed in Fig. 9.3. This particular schematic illustrates that the colposcopist could see the whole transformation zone, has identified a significant lesion within it and also identified that some areas may be worse than others (although as both are preinvasive this would not alter the treatment strategy). Had atypical vessels or an irregular surface contour been documented then a colposcopic opinion of early invasion might have been made.

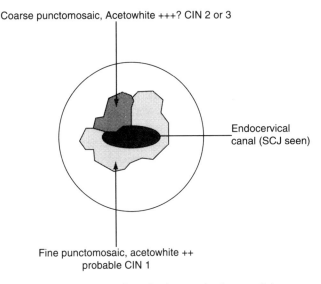

Coarse punctomosaic, Acetowhite +++? CIN 2 or 3

Endocervical
canal (SCJ seen)

Fine punctomosaic, acetowhite ++
probable CIN 1

Fig. 9.3 Diagrammatic representation of colposcopic abnormalities.

The shortcomings of this method are that it is difficult to quantify the size of abnormality and is wholly subjective and difficult to reproduce. The former can be partly addressed by attempting to semiquantitate the lesion. This can be done by superimposing imaginary lines on the image so as to divide the cervix into 'measurement sectors'. First, a circle is drawn on the cervix with its centre at the middle of the external os and its radius reaching to a point midway between the external os and the cervicovaginal junction (line A). A second line bisects the cervix laterally (line B) and a third antero-posteriorly (line C). In this way the cervix is divided into eight sectors (figure 4). There are consistent data linking large-surface-area lesions with high-grade histology and also an increased likelihood of treatment failure (Fig. 9.4).

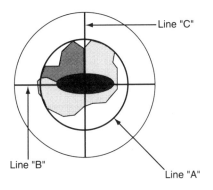

Line "C"

Line "B"

Line "A"

Fig. 9.4 Schematic of a '5 sector' lesion.

Freehand drawing is also used to illustrate abnormalities at the vaginal vault. If the cervix is still in place this is usually represented by just extending the area of abnormality on to the vagina, as indicated in Fig. 9.5.

Sometimes, after a hysterectomy for preinvasive disease a woman may persist in having, or develop, abnormal vaginal vault smears. This might indicate vaginal intraepithelial neoplasia. In this situation the vaginal vault is usually pictured as in Fig. 9.6. The transverse line represents the vaginal vault scar and the angled lines at either end represent the vaginal angles. This is not very satisfactory, as the vaginal angles can be deeply pocketed following hysterectomy and the schematic cannot account for this.

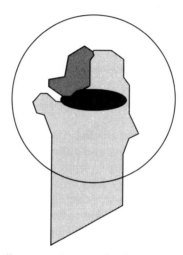

Fig. 9.5 Lesion extending on to the posterior fornix.

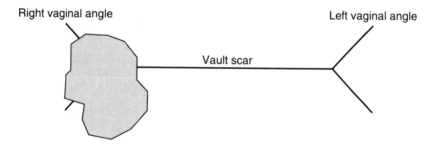

Fig. 9.6 Lesion involving the right vaginal angle and the vaginal vault scar.

OTHER METHODS OF IMAGE CAPTURE AND STORAGE

Colpophotography

Photography offers an obvious solution to the problem of subjectivity and accuracy. Most colposcopes will allow for the attachment of a beam-splitting device so that the image seen by the colposcopist can be diverted to a fixed camera without altering the image seen. There is usually some loss of light intensity. The camera is attached directly to the beam-splitter and no lens adjustments are necessary once the equipment has been set up. The film used is 35 mm colour film (usual speed ASA 200), with flash exposure on an f16/32 aperture setting. Using this set-up limits the depth of focus, which is the major problem of colpophotography. Black and white film is preferred, with the addition of a green filter if the subepithelial capillary architecture is to be emphasized (good for atypical vessels). A flash device may be used: a ring flash around the colposcope objective lens is useful in this situation.

Photographs may also be taken without the use of the colposcope. Hand-held cameras have to be used at higher shutter speeds to compensate for shake. Again a flash device is necessary and in addition some alternative light source to illuminate the cervix to enable the target shot to be focused properly. The quality of these photographs is generally inferior to those taken with the aid of the colposcope.

A further development of photography was the introduction of the cerviscope. This consists of a 35 mm camera body, a 50 mm extension ring and a 100 mm macrolens with ring strobe light. This in effect is a customized camera of fixed focal length that takes 35 mm exposures under enhanced illumination and flash capacity. Since the exposure time is determined by the duration of the flash of the strobe light (less than 1/2000th of a second), hand vibrations of the person holding the cerviscope will not affect the quality of the slides. The device was primarily intended as a substitute for colposcopy (in areas where no colposcopy was available). The exposures taken are sent for expert analysis (by projection and analysis at a fixed distance from the screen), thus enabling selection of those women who would require colposcopy and biopsy.

All the above photographic methods of image capture have similar drawbacks.

1. The image is not immediately available for scrutiny; therefore the eventual quality of the image cannot be assessed.
2. The cervix is a three-dimensional structure, whereas colpophotographs are not (even with enhanced depth of focus this is a potential shortcoming)
3. Transparencies are a less than ideal method of storing image data alongside other data.
4. It is relatively expensive.
5. Once collected, the image cannot be enhanced, magnified or annotated.

Videocolposcopy

Modern video cameras are small and produce high-quality images (particularly three-chip cameras). These can also be attached, via a beam-splitting device, to a standard colposcope. Many clinics routinely employ video for patient information purposes (although not all patients wish to observe procedures) and for teaching. Because video offers a time dimension as well as the image, several different views of the same cervix are possible and can all be stored. Views include different magnifications, addition of green filters, before and after the application of saline, acetic acid or iodine. One video, therefore, can contain the same information as multiple still exposures.

Video images can be stored on tape or disc. The former is both bulky and inconvenient in terms of recall. The latter only suffers from problems of memory, i.e. video images require large amounts of computer storage such that one standard 3.5 in floppy disc can only store three or four compressed video images. Compact disc offers greater scope for image storage but is more expensive.

Images captured by video cameras are digitized signals. Utilizing this allows for both storage and image manipulation. Some colposcopy clinics already employ digitized image capture, storage and analysis and it is proving to be a useful teaching, audit and research tool. Whether it actually enhances clinical care is debatable.

The computer's storage, analysis and manipulation systems allow the images to be instantly recalled, compared to previously recalled images, enhanced in terms of contrast, sharpness and brightness. Additionally, 'electronic' filters can be employed to selectively enhance vasculature, acetowhiteness, etc. As the image is stored it can also be electronically measured (area, perimeter), thus dispensing with the need for semiquantitative measurements. Hard copy of the image can be produced to store alongside the patient's written record or, alternatively, the written information can be stored in a database alongside the stored image, allowing for a complete set of electronic notes.

Few clinics have this capacity as yet and it is arguable that few will actually need this high degree of data management. Nevertheless, a structured and meticulous approach to data management in the colposcopy clinic, be it handwritten structured case notes or direct-entry computerized notes, is and will continue to be an important aspect of work in the colposcopy clinic and is a discipline that should be acquired by all practising colposcopists.

LEARNING POINTS

1. Accurate recording of the information gained at colposcopy is an important aspect of service provision.
2. Minimum datasets need not record information on previous sexual history unless this is part of an ethically agreed protocol or is part of a genito-urinary medicine service.
3. Electronic storage of information will allow for the automation of repetitive tasks such as appointment scheduling and communication with referring agencies. It will also allow fail-safes to be built into the system to track invasive cancers, defaulting patients, etc.
4. Image recording is useful for making comparisons at further clinic visits. The simplest methods, such as hand-drawings, are also the least objective.
5. Objective image-capturing techniques include various photographic and videocolposcopic techniques.

MCQS

23. Recording information in colposcopy clinics:
    a. When taking a history from a patient with an abnormal cervical smear it is important to ask about the age at first intercourse
    b. All patients having colposcopy should have a bimanual examination
    c. Invagination of the vaginal angles following hysterectomy makes image recording difficult
    d. It is unnecessary to record a gynaecological history at the time of colposcopy
    e. The use of digital image capture has no proven benefits in managing patients in the colposcopy clinic

24. In colpophotography:
    a. Hand-held 35 mm cameras give poorer quality photographs than those taken through the colposcope
    b. Black and white film (enhanced by the addition of a green filter) is better for recording vascular architecture
    c. Videophotography gives better depth of focus than still photography
    d. Cervicographs are assessed by an expert, who examines the final colour print of the cervix
    e. An objective lens of 400 mm is ideal for photographing the cervix

Conservative management of CIN

M. I. Shafi

BACKGROUND

There is a large discrepancy between the number of women with abnormal cervical cytology and those developing invasive cervical cancer. Mortality associated with cervical cancer continues to fall, with a 15% decrease between 1985 and 1991. This compares with an increasing number of women having cytological abnormalities of which only a minority will develop invasive cancer. The invasive potential of CIN has been known for a long time. However, trying to quantify the risk overall and especially for the individual woman is fraught with danger. In some studies, the progression rates are extremely high, with almost all high-grade lesions progressing to invasive cancer, and in others only a small minority will progress. What is known is that the more severe the cytological abnormality, the higher the risk of finding invasive disease when the woman is assessed. Similarly, a group of women with a histological diagnosis of CIN 3 are more likely to progress than a group of women with CIN 1 or HPV-associated changes only. However, this does not help in predicting for the individual woman her risk for progression from CIN to invasive cancer. Based partly on these facts, the Royal College of Obstetricians and Gynaecologists (RCOG) recommendations in 1987 stated that all grades of CIN should undergo treatment. More recently it has been realized that this policy has led to overtreatment for many women, especially with the

Handbook of Colposcopy, edited by David Luesley, Mahmood Shafi and Joe Jordan. Published in 1996 by Chapman & Hall, London. ISBN 0 412 71550 3

introduction of a 'see and treat' management strategy using large loop excision of the transformation zone (LLETZ). Reviewing the evidence, the national guidelines were changed in 1992 to state that CIN 1 may be treated or kept under close surveillance.

HOW DO WE SELECT PATIENTS?

In many units, the women are assessed in colposcopy units and colposcopically directed punch biopsies are taken from the worst area of abnormality. Dependent upon the results of this, the woman is either offered treatment or observation as indicated. For the high-grade lesions (CIN 2 and 3) immediate treatment should be conducted. For the low-grade lesions (CIN 1 or HPV-associated changes), treatment may be offered or a deferred management strategy may be adopted depending on the circumstances. For example, in a woman who is 45 and has completed her family, a punch biopsy diagnosis of CIN 1 is likely to lead to treatment. Someone in her early 20s with the same diagnosis who is nulliparous and has only a small area of abnormality may be offered a conservative management option in the hope that the lesion will regress over time and both colposcopic assessment and cervical cytology will return to normal.

In other centres, it is normal practice not to take any diagnostic punch biopsies prior to treatment. In these units, a colposcopic diagnosis on the grounds of abnormal cervical cytology is deemed sufficient, but this is affected by the subjective nature of colposcopic assessment. There may be considerable inter- as well as intraobserver disagreement in relation to the colposcopic findings. These units mostly practise excisional forms of treatment (LLETZ, laser excision) and the excised transformation zone is sent for histological diagnosis. Some women will not require treatment, among whom will be women who have abnormal cervical cytology and no colposcopic abnormality. In these, colposcopic and cytological review should continue until at least two negative smears are obtained 6 months apart before discharging the woman back to her general practitioner. In those women deemed to have a low-grade lesion on colposcopic assessment, a deferred management strategy may be adopted only if the colposcopist is confident of the diagnosis. Treatment should be offered if the lesion worsens either because the cytology shows more severe changes or because colposcopically the lesion appears worse (e.g. the size of the lesion increases or stigmata of high-grade disease, such as coarse mosaicism, become apparent). Not taking a colposcopically directed biopsy may be perceived as an inaccurate science, but so could taking a directed biopsy from the wrong area of a lesion. Those with sufficient experience are normally happy to rely on the colposcopic assessment for those women thought to have a low-grade lesion, as review cytology and colposcopy will pick up any progression of the lesion.

HISTOLOGICAL INTERPRETATION

While taking a punch biopsy would seem judicious if there is concern about the diagnosis, one has to be aware that histological interpretation is not without its problems. While there is good agreement at the higher end of the CIN spectrum, this is not so at the lower end when trying to differentiate CIN 1 and HPV-associated changes. There is also a tendency to overcall low-grade lesions on punch biopsy, leading to unnecessary treatment. Further bias may be introduced if the worst area of colposcopic abnormality is not sampled by the colposcopist.

PROGRESSIVE POTENTIAL OF CIN

The pathological spectrum of CIN has been arbitrarily divided into three grades: 1, 2 and 3 (Chapter 3). These grades are associated with a different risk of progressive potential and have recently been revised to high-grade lesions (CIN 2, 3) that are likely to be cancer precursors and low-grade lesions (CIN 1 and HPV-associated changes) that have unknown but probable low risk of progressive potential. The progressive potential of CIN is also likely to be related to the size of the lesion as well as its grade. For example, a large CIN 3 lesion would be expected to have a higher risk of progression than a small focus of CIN 3 surrounded by a low-grade lesion. Despite this, there is unanimity that once CIN 3 is diagnosed, treatment should be offered. An exception to this would be in the pregnant woman, where treatment may need to be deferred (Chapter 15).

DEFERRED MANAGEMENT

If a decision is made between the colposcopist and the woman to defer treatment for a low-grade lesion, sufficient stress needs to be placed on the need for continued colposcopic and cytological surveillance. If there is any likelihood of non-compliance, then treatment should be offered. For those willing to comply, both colposcopy and cytology should be repeated at 6-monthly intervals. If the abnormality persists either colposcopically or cytologically (usually an arbitrary upper limit of 24 months is set), then treatment should be offered. If the lesion regresses, the surveillance is continued until two consecutive smears are negative, at which point the woman may be returned to the 3-yearly screening programme.

THE PROBLEM OF DEFAULT

This is an area of considerable concern in those women undergoing deferred management. In two recent prospective studies looking at the management of minor cytological abnormalities, the cumulative default rate is approximately 20%. Depending on the catchment area of the colposcopy clinic this may be as high as 30%. If there is a problem of default from clinics in those women selected for deferred management, then this policy is not sustainable and should be abandoned for a more pragmatic approach. If, however, default rates are low with a stable population, a selective policy of deferred management can be safely undertaken without prejudicing the long-term prognosis for the woman. Mechanisms should exist in all colposcopy clinics to limit the problem of default and this might consist of better communication with the women concerned, a better environment in the colposcopy clinics, explanation as to why compliance is important, clinic times that are suitable for women with varying commitments (e.g. evening clinics) and appropriate counselling. A key element is that all advice given to the women should be the same irrespective of the source, and in this respect written instructions and advice are extremely useful (Chapter 17).

SUMMARY

While the conservative option in the management of CIN is not suitable for all cases, it is certainly one to consider if we are to impact on the overtreatment potential of a 'see and treat' strategy that has currently found favour amongst UK colposcopists. This is particularly the case for younger women with low-grade lesions, as many of these will regress over time. During any conservative management strategy, the importance of compliance with the surveillance programme cannot be overstressed. The management algorithm (Fig. 10.1) summarizes a conservative approach to the management of mildly abnormal smears.

LEARNING POINTS

1. Not all cases of CIN will progress to invasive cancer.
2. High-grade CIN is known to have malignant potential whereas low-grade lesions have unknown malignant potential.
3. Accurate colposcopic assessment and appropriate directed biopsies are necessary for those women considered suitable for conservative management.
4. High-grade lesions should be treated once diagnosed.
5. Low-grade lesions can either be treated or kept under close surveillance.
6. Default rates should be considered when deciding whether a woman may be conservatively managed.

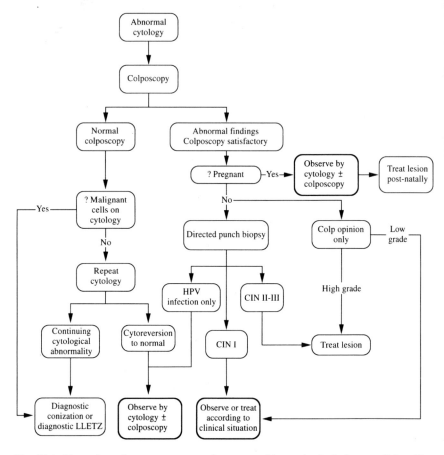

Fig. 10.1 Flow chart for management of women with cytological abnormalities. (Reproduced with permission from RCOG Yearbook, 1995, RCOG Press).

MCQS

25. Epidemiology:
    a. The overall age incidence of cervical cancer is increasing
    b. Cervical cancer is the commonest female cancer
    c. Approximately 7% of all cervical smears taken are abnormal to some degree
    d. The commonest cytological abnormality is severe dyskaryosis
    e. Almost 5.5 million smears are performed annually in the UK

26. Patient selection:
    a. All cases of CIN must undergo immediate treatment

b. Colposcopic opinion alone may not be enough if conservative management is being considered
c. A directed punch biopsy will always give an accurate assessment of the degree of abnormality
d. CIN in pregnancy should be immediately treated
e. Age is a consideration in the management of low-grade lesions

27. Non-treatment of cytological abnormalities:
   a. If there is no lesion present at colposcopy and the cervical smear is normal a woman can safely be returned to the call and recall scheme
   b. Women with CIN 1 have a lower progressive potential than those with CIN 3
   c. HPV-associated lesions can be easily distinguished from CIN 1 on colposcopy
   d. HPV-associated changes are easily distinguished from CIN 1 on histological examination
   e. CIN has a centripetal distribution (i.e. higher-grade CIN is centrally placed in a lesion)

28. Colposcopy in pregnancy:
   a. Colposcopy and cervical smears may cause a miscarriage in early pregnancy
   b. Colposcopy is made easier in pregnancy due to hormonal effects on the cervix
   c. A punch biopsy is taken if CIN is suspected colposcopically
   d. Treatment of CIN may be deferred until the postnatal period
   e. If invasion is suspected, a wedge biopsy is taken for diagnostic purposes under general anaesthesia

29. Deferred management:
   a. Default rates may have an influence on deferred treatment strategies
   b. A transient population should be offered immediate treatment once CIN is diagnosed
   c. Peak incidence of low-grade lesions is between 35 and 40 years
   d. Stress levels return to normal immediately if the woman is offered deferred management
   e. The stress of colposcopy is similar to that of major surgery

D. M. Luesley

INTRODUCTION

Any screening programme must have as one of its components an intervention that is timely and effective in preventing the natural progression of disease. In CIN, this intervention or treatment occurs following the cytological, colposcopic and histological recognition of precursors that carry an increased risk of progression to invasive disease.

Not all CIN will become cancer. There is therefore a need to select cases for treatment on the basis of risk. Once a decision to treat has been made, the most appropriate form of treatment is selected.

WHO REQUIRES TREATMENT?

There is a growing body of opinion which feels that minor abnormalities (CIN 1 with or without koilocytosis, or koilocytosis alone) may be observed as there is a reasonable prospect of spontaneous resolution over time. The critical issue here is one of accurate initial diagnosis. Up to 40% of minor cytological abnormalities will be associated with underlying high-grade disease and as most if not all colposcopists would recommend treatment of high-grade lesions, decisions that rely on cytology alone will significantly underestimate such lesions.

Handbook of Colposcopy, edited by David Luesley, Mahmood Shafi and Joe Jordan. Published in 1996 by Chapman & Hall, London. ISBN 0 412 71550 3

The addition of colposcopy improves the selection process yet is still not 100% accurate. Even adding directed or targeted biopsies fails to achieve this level of accuracy in diagnosis. Given the inadequacies of our diagnostic procedures we are left in a situation where specificity is sacrificed in favour of sensitivity, i.e. it is more acceptable to overtreat a group of women who might never have developed cancer in order not to miss the smaller group who might well progress. This philosophy is possible only because the available treatment modalities are relatively simple, safe and effective. Thus the treatment methodology itself is a variable that determines the level of intervention. As an example, if the only treatment method available was radical hysterectomy then the threshold for offering treatment would be much higher. At the other extreme, simple outpatient loop excision, which is quick, safe, cheap and effective, has resulted in a lowering of the intervention threshold, a practice typified by the 'see and treat' philosophy.

'SEE AND TREAT'

The true 'see and treat' approach is one that assumes that all women referred to a colposcopy clinic with an abnormal smear are at an increased risk of developing cancer and are therefore treated by an excisional method at their first attendance to the clinic. The advantages of such an approach are as follows.

1. All patients at risk are treated.
2. There is a more rapid return to cytological normality.
3. All occult cancers will be detected.
4. There are fewer visits required therefore less cost to service and patient.
5. Very little if any colposcopic expertise is required.

These points may seem convincing yet this approach leads to a massive amount of 'over-intervention'. Even though the morbidity associated with loop excision is low it is not nil; therefore unnecessary morbidity will be generated. Some would argue that this type of early and effective intervention will be associated with a lesser degree of psychosocial trauma. This has yet to be confirmed and the converse may also be true, i.e. the very act of intervention reinforces the 'disease state'. While many clinics currently do employ a 'see and treat' approach, more are adopting the more conservative 'select and treat' philosophy.

'SELECT AND TREAT'

This aims to reduce overtreatment. Based upon the cytological status, colposcopic appearances of the lesion and if necessary targeted biopsies, the colposcopist aims only to treat those where there is a reasonable suspicion of high-grade disease. Naturally some will still be overtreated and there is an additional burden of counselling and following up those who have not been treated. A higher level of colposcopic expertise is required and it is less efficient in resource use. As diagnostic acumen improves, particularly as we employ specific tests of outcome such as the possible use of HPV subtyping, the selection process will become more refined.

Some of the criteria employed in constructing the treatment algorithm are shown in Fig. 11.1.

Cytology and colposcopy follow-up are integral components of a 'select and treat' strategy and, although there are no data to suggest how long such a follow-up period should be, an arbitrary figure of 2 years is usually employed. Few women will be happy to undertake further surveillance, particularly if their smear remains abnormal albeit a minor abnormality, furthermore, those who have had persistently abnormal smears for this period of time are

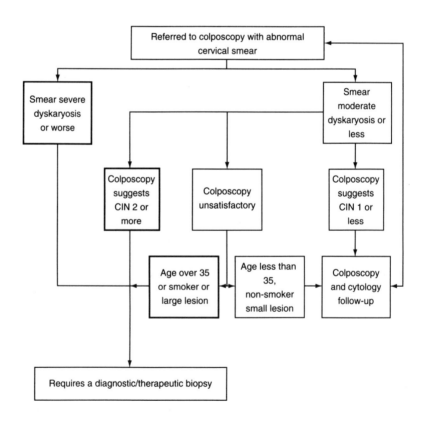

Fig. 11.1 Who to select for diagnostic/therapeutic biopsy.

more likely to have a lesion that will not regress. This, however, is an area for further research.

If, either at the first visit or during subsequent follow-up, the criteria for intervention are met, a further series of decisions based upon the three criteria (cytology, colposcopy and histology) is required (Fig. 11.2).

The types of treatment available are many and individual choices should be matched against specific criteria. Perhaps the most important decision to make at this point is to exclude invasive disease.

EXCLUDING INVASIVE DISEASE

Local destruction or excision are inappropriate methods to manage invasive disease although some cases of stage Ia1 and Ia2 disease can be managed by large cones (knife, loop or laser). Invasive disease should be suspected if:

1. naked eye examination is suspicious;
2. colposcopy is suspicious of invasion (atypical vessels, irregular cervix, etc.);

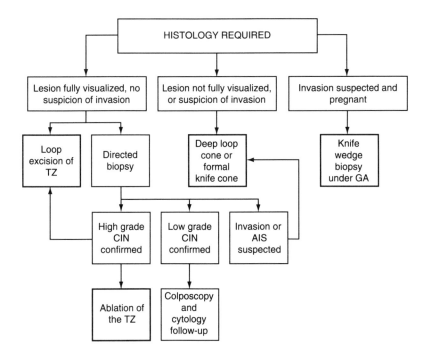

Fig. 11.2 Selection of biopsy method.

3. cytological features of invasion (malignant diathesis);
4. malignant glandular cells in the smear;
5. the whole transformation zone cannot be visualized; in this situation colposcopy is deemed unsatisfactory as there will always be the possibility of an invasive process within the part of the TZ that has not been seen.

If any of these criteria are met then a large representative biopsy of the whole transformation zone should be taken. The methods employed to achieve this are:

1. knife cone biopsy;
2. deep loop cone biopsy;
3. laser cone biopsy.

Most would still favour a knife cone in these situations as there is less likelihood of damaging the excision margins. Clear interpretation of the excision margins is important for accurate substaging as it is impossible to substage stage Ia cancers unless the whole lesion is seen in the specimen. This may not be possible if there is any degree of thermal artefact obscuring interpretation of the cone edges.

If adenocarcinoma in situ is suspected, the management should be as for suspected invasive disease.

Suspected invasion in pregnancy

In pregnancy, biopsies are usually avoided because of the increased risk of haemorrhage. They are therefore only performed if there is a high degree of suspicion of an invasive process. This is obviously an area where expert colposcopy is required. To minimize cervical trauma and damage, yet still provide adequate histological material to allow an accurate diagnosis of invasion or no invasion, a compromise is made and a wedge of the most atypical part of the TZ is removed under general anaesthesia. This must be regarded as diagnostic only and is not a form of treatment for invasion or CIN.

THE PRINCIPLES OF TREATING CIN

Several basic principles apply to all forms of treatment.

1. If CIN is to be treated, all grades are treated in the same way. High-grade CIN does not require any more radicality than low-grade CIN.
2. The whole transformation zone should be treated or excised and not just the area where CIN has been identified.
3. CIN can and does involve gland crypts, therefore any treatment form must

address this issue and treat to below the level of gland crypts. A minimum depth of destruction of 7 mm is recommended.
4. All treated patients remain at a slightly increased risk of cancer in the future. Cervical cytology follow-up should be offered to all treated patients.

TYPES OF TREATMENT

Many types of treatment are available and they fall into one of two categories. These are excisional methods where the TZ is removed intact and therefore available for full histological assessment, and destructive or ablative methods. In the latter, histological diagnosis must always be obtained by biopsy before treatment is applied. This is the only way to reduce the risk of inadvertently treating invasive disease. It therefore follows that if a 'see and treat' policy is to be used, an excisional form of treatment must be employed (Table 11.1).

The difference between a cone biopsy and a TZ excision is largely a matter of degree. Cone biopsy usually refers to a procedure where an attempt is made to remove at least two-thirds of the endocervical canal, occasionally more. A TZ excision refers to a procedure where the TZ can be seen and the excision process purely aims at obtaining the correct depth (> 7 mm) and reasonable clearance (> 3 mm) at the edges.

Cryocautery is becoming less popular, largely as a result of published results indicating higher failure rates. This of course, may not be the fault of the technique but of the operator. Nevertheless it is probably less effective in achieving the appropriate depth of destruction and can be difficult with large lesions.

Chemodestructive techniques have been performed but the long-term outcomes are poor and they are not used in clinical practice now.

Cold coagulation is really a misnomer. A probe, similar to a cryoprobe, is applied to the cervix but the tissue is destroyed by heat (> 120°C).

Hysterectomy is an effective form of treatment but is only used if there is an indication for the procedure on its own, i.e. confirmed CIN but also a complaint of menorrhagia or some other problem that would be best managed by hysterectomy. As with the other forms of treatment it is important to

Table 11.1 Treatment methods

Excisional	Destructive
Knife cone biopsy	Cryocautery
Laser cone biopsy	Laser ablation
Loop cone biopsy	Electrodiathermy
Laser or loop TZ excision	Cold coagulation
Hysterectomy	Chemodestruction (5FU, DNCB)

exclude invasion first as a simple hysterectomy would be inappropriate treatment for invasive disease. Furthermore, if hysterectomy is the chosen method of treatment, colposcopy should accurately delineate the most caudal extension of the TZ in order to include any vaginal extension in a vaginal cuff.

ANALGESIA

Treatment can be performed on an outpatient basis, usually with a local anaesthetic. The cervix is infiltrated with a mixture of a local anaesthetic (lignocaine, prilocaine) and a vasoconstrictor (octapressin or adrenaline). A dental syringe and needle are employed and the cervix infiltrated to a point where the tissues are seen to blanche. Care should be taken to infiltrate around and not into the TZ as there is a theoretical risk that malignant cells could be introduced deep into the stroma. Local anaesthetics are usually effective in two minutes and allow most of the outpatient excisional and ablative procedures to be completed with minimal if any discomfort to the patient.

The following procedures can be performed as outpatients under local analgesia:

1. Laser ablation
2. Cold coagulation
3. Loop and laser excision.

Cryocautery can be performed without any analgesia.

Some patients will be better treated under a general anaesthetic. It is obvious that hysterectomy should be performed under a general anaesthetic, as indeed are most formal knife cones and wedge biopsies. About 10% of women, however, will be better managed under a GA by one of the outpatient techniques. This is because of patient anxiety or request or because of poor access to the cervix. In the latter, better access and control can be achieved in the anaesthetized patient.

COMPLICATIONS OF TREATMENT

Immediate

Pain and haemorrhage are the two problems that are likely to occur. The former affects very few women now that most treatments are performed under local anaesthetic. Significant haemorrhage, sufficient to either prolong treatment or require remedial measures such as suturing, admission, etc., is quite uncommon (less than 2% of all cases). In most cases bleeding can be controlled either with the laser or by diathermy. Cold coagulation does not cause primary haemorrhage. There is no reliable way of predicting who will haemorrhage. Obvious infections such as *Trichomonas vaginalis* should be treated prior to local excision or ablation as they are associated with increased cervical vascularity. It used to be thought that treatment should not be performed either during or shortly after a period. Apart from the more obvious problems of achieving good visibility, menstruation is not associated with any increased haemorrhagic morbidity.

Delayed

Secondary haemorrhage can occur any time up to 14 days and is usually the result of a minor infection in the crater where the TZ had existed. This will occur in 1–2% of treated patients. Prophylactic antibiotics are used in some clinics but their use has not been shown to reduce the frequency of this complication.

Pelvic infection has been reported following local cervical treatment but only on an *ad hoc* basis. There would appear to be an increased risk of this if an intrauterine device is fitted immediately following treatment.

Cervical stenosis (defined as narrowing of the external os to less than 3 mm) occurs after all methods of treatment. It is much more likely to occur after large conizations and affects 1–2% of women managed by loop excision of the transformation zone. The complication is more likely in postmenopausal women. Cervical stenosis may be asymptomatic or cause dysmenorrhoea or, in extreme cases, haematometra. The anatomical distortion of the cervix may make follow-up cervical cytology either difficult or inaccurate as the new TZ may become inaccessible.

There are no data confirming that local destruction or excision result in reduced fertility, although this is a natural concern and theoretical possibility. There are no data suggesting either an increase in miscarriage, preterm labour or failure of the cervix to dilate in labour. Some groups have however noted a poorer obstetric performance in treated women. Whether this relates to direct complications of treatment or perhaps to pre-existing factors such as smoking is uncertain. While largely unconfirmed, the concerns over possible impairment of reproductive performance are sufficient to provide support for a more selective approach to treatment.

TREATMENT OUTCOMES

Most methods of treatment have success rates in the order of 95%. Not all patients return to cytological normality within 6 months but very few, if managed appropriately, will have persisting CIN. The incidence of invasive cancer following local treatments is similar for all methods, including hysterectomy.

CONCLUSIONS

Treatment is an integral part of the programme for the prevention of cervical cancer. Treatment should not be undertaken by anyone other than trained colposcopists. With careful selection for treatment and appropriate use of treatment methods successful outcomes with low morbidity can be achieved.

LEARNING POINTS

1. Not all patients with CIN will require treatment, although most with high-grade disease will.
2. It is important to exclude invasion prior to local destruction.
3. 'See and treat' management should only be performed using excisional treatment methods.
4. Most methods of local treatment can be performed under local anaesthetic and have success rates in excess of 90%
5. If there is any suspicion of invasion, large representative biopsies should be taken.
6. Only trained colposcopists should undertake treatment.
7. Hysterectomy is appropriate treatment if there is a specific indication. It does not dispense with the need for a thorough colposcopic evaluation first.
8. Although good data are lacking relating treatment to impaired reproductive performance, there are sufficient concerns to be more selective about treatment.

MCQS

30. In the treatment of CIN:
    a. CIN 3 requires more radical treatment than CIN 1
    b. Colposcopy is required before any treatment method
    c. Before ablation, a directed biopsy should be performed
    d. Laser vaporization can be used to 'see and treat' without recourse to biopsy
    e. Local anaesthetic is not required for outpatient loop excision

31. The following are recognized complications of diathermy loop excision:
    a. Haemorrhage
    b. Pelvic inflammatory disease
    c. Cervical stenosis
    d. Infertility
    e. Dyspareunia

32. Treatment of CIN should not be performed:
    a. In pregnancy
    b. If there is an acute vaginal infection
    c. In the luteal phase
    d. During menstruation
    e. In women who are HIV-positive

12 | Follow-up after colposcopy

H. Kitchener

INTRODUCTION

Appropriate follow-up is an essential part of any colposcopy management protocol. The purpose of this chapter is to explain the need for follow-up in both treated and untreated patients. The methods of follow-up which should be employed and for how long will also be discussed. Colposcopic examination is employed in a variety of clinical situations:

1. as the initial means of diagnosis following an abnormal smear;
2. as a means of selective ablation or excision of the transformation zone;
3. as a means of follow-up after treatment of CIN;
4. continued surveillance following an inconclusive initial examination.

THE NEED FOR FOLLOW-UP AFTER TREATMENT OF CIN

The reasons why follow-up is so important following treatment are threefold:

1. to ensure that there is no residual CIN, or even cancer;
2. to ensure that any recurrence of CIN is detected;
3. to ensure that there have been no clinical problems since treatment.

In order to design the most effective follow-up protocol it is necessary to have an understanding both of the risks of treatment failure and of longer-term recurrence of both CIN and cancer. The more rigorous the follow-up protocol, the less likely that treatment failure will go unrecognized. On the other hand,

Handbook of Colposcopy, edited by David Luesley, Mahmood Shafi and Joe Jordan. Published in 1996 by Chapman & Hall, London. ISBN 0 412 71550 3

a more intensive protocol will consume more clinical resources, and women may be made to experience continued anxiety. For some women the process of treatment is not over until discharge from the colposcopy clinic and until that time there may be continued concern.

It is now widely accepted that primary treatment of CIN should have a success rate of 90–95% for the majority of cases where the SCJ is visible. This high figure would not apply to CIN where a cone biopsy was required because of disease extending into the canal. Under these circumstances it is difficult to ensure adequate excision at the endocervical margin. Risk factors for treatment failure include: large lesions; CIN 3; older patients; incomplete excision margins; operative difficulties during treatment, e.g. poor access; and bleeding. Follow-up in such cases needs to be particularly thorough.

TREATMENT FAILURE

The term 'treatment failure' is intended to cover both residual disease, resulting from inadequate ablation or incomplete excision, and recurring disease. At which point we can strictly distinguish between residual disease and disease recurrence is a moot point. Disease that is identified 2 years following treatment, with normal cytology between times, is likely to be recurrence. In most cases this will have resulted from progressive enlargement of a residual focus, but in a few cases this will be a true re-occurrence, i.e. a new second lesion in the regenerated transformation zone. Whether or not treated women are at increased risk of developing a new lesion, compared with the general population, is not known. For practical purposes it is sufficient to say that the risk remains, and therefore continued cytological screening is essential.

LENGTH OF FOLLOW-UP

Some insight into the pattern of treatment can be gained from a large study carried out in our department. We identified a 94% success rate following over 2000 laser ablations for CIN. Out of the 119 treatment failures, 70% were identified within the first 12 months, 24% in the second 12 months and only 6% thereafter. This pattern probably reflects the three categories of treatment failure described previously. Follow-up during the first 12 months will generally identify truly residual disease. The second 12 months will largely identify residual foci which have enlarged and become detectable and the very small number of cases identified thereafter may well be true new lesions. This pattern of recurrence indicates the need for a more intensive period of follow-up during the first 12 months followed by a second phase of less intensive follow-up prior to returning to normal screening. Protocols vary, but a typical regime would be two checks in the first year, annual checks until 5 years and return to routine screening thereafter.

METHOD OF FOLLOW-UP

The next consideration is the role that colposcopy has in the follow-up of treated patients. Cytology is the mainstay, with the need for colposcopy being more debatable. The obvious advantage of colposcopy is that of a safety net in the event of a false-negative smear, which can occur partly because residual lesions may be very small. One of the problems of colposcopy following treatment is that regenerating epithelium can sometimes resemble CIN, because a rather prominent vascular pattern may be seen in the new transformation zone. In the previously mentioned follow-up study from Aberdeen, 20% of residual lesions were identified colposcopically in the presence of normal cytology. These lesions would probably have been detected cytologically over time but early diagnosis has the advantage of identifying the need for a second treatment prior to discharge from the colposcopy clinic. A follow-up study from Newcastle has suggested that cytology is perfectly adequate for follow-up. The national guidelines accept that while colposcopy is optional for follow-up it may improve early diagnosis. In a recently performed survey of colposcopy practice in the UK the majority of clinics reported the use of both colposcopy and cytology on at least one occasion.

Follow-up routines

A typical follow-up protocol would be as follows:

1. **First post-treatment assessment:** Colposcopy clinic at 6 months, for colposcopy and cytology;
2. **Primary care (general practice):** Annually from 12 months–5 years – cytology.

Thereafter the women would return to routine recall.

Following treatment, the squamocolumnar junction (SCJ) usually remains visible. Sometimes the SCJ remains well up the canal, rendering colposcopy unsatisfactory and of little value. Under these circumstances many will employ endocervical cytology with an instrument such as the Cytobrush. If this is to be employed it is better to colposcope first because the endocervical brush usually causes bleeding, which can obscure the view the colposcopist has of the ectocervix.

THE PROBLEM OF DEFAULT

One important practical difficulty of follow-up is that of the women who default. These women are at increased risk of eventually developing cancer and a protocol must be in place to ensure that continued efforts are made to follow up. If the patient defaults once, a reminder should be sent. If she persists in defaulting the best approach is to assume she no longer wishes to attend the colposcopy clinic and to try to ensure follow-up smears by the general practitioner. It is important to stress the necessity of follow-up at the time that treatment is carried out.

INVASIVE CANCER FOLLOWING TREATMENT OF CIN

Invasive cancer is the ultimate form of treatment failure after a diagnosis of CIN. If it is detected within 12 months of treatment, it is likely that there was early cancer present at the time of treatment. Microinvasive disease may be missed by an inexpert colposcopist and incompletely ablated by conservative treatment. The quoted risk of frankly invasive cancer following treatment of CIN is around 1 in 1000 and, in addition, 1 in 1000 will be diagnosed with microinvasion. It is almost inevitable that the occasional very early invasive lesion will be inappropriately treated by conservative therapy and this probably accounts for the majority of such cases. It is possible that the increasing use of excisional therapy will reduce the number of invasive cases, because the occasional colposcopically undiagnosed microinvasive lesion may well be identified histologically in a diathermy-loop-excised specimen, thus ensuring appropriate treatment. As the incidence of invasive disease falls as a result of improved screening, these cases diagnosed after treatment assume increasing importance.

FOLLOW-UP AFTER HYSTERECTOMY

Normally the 15–20 % of women who undergo a hysterectomy for reasons unrelated to CIN are removed from the screening programme. This arrangement is altered if CIN is involved. There are three situations where CIN needs to be considered.

1. in women who had treatment of CIN in the past and subsequently underwent a hysterectomy for an unrelated indication with no CIN present.
2. where a hysterectomy is performed for an unrelated indication but CIN is an incidental finding.
3. where a hysterectomy is performed as the treatment for persistent CIN or abnormal smears.

In general, provided the hysterectomy specimen in the first scenario does not contain CIN no follow-up is required. In scenarios 2 and 3, when CIN is present in the hysterectomy specimen the correct measure is to undertake colposcopy of the healed vault to ensure there is no residual intraepithelial neoplasia and, if none is present, to undertake cytology of the vault (Chapter 14).

CLINICAL PROBLEMS FOLLOWING COLPOSCOPIC TREATMENT

In general the treatment of CIN involves little morbidity, but at the first follow-up visit an enquiry should be made about any symptoms experienced. It is not uncommon for women to mention some discomfort and irregular bleeding for a few weeks following treatment, but this usually resolves with time. Occasionally dysmenorrhoea is experienced and cervical stenosis should be sought, which is said to occur in 1–2% of cases. Sometimes cervical stenosis is seen at colposcopy in the absence of significant symptoms (Chapter 15).

FOLLOW-UP COLPOSCOPY AFTER FAILURE TO DIAGNOSE CIN

In cases of mild and moderate dyskaryosis, colposcopy may not reveal an obvious lesion. If this occurs with a normal repeat smear then it is reasonable to conclude that CIN is not present and to discharge the patient. If, however, the repeat smear is again abnormal, it is best to repeat colposcopy at a visit in 3–6 months. If the cytology continues to be abnormal in the absence of an obvious lesion it is permissible to treat the cervix, preferably by excision. This will encourage a return to normal cytology. Yet another scenario is when a directed biopsy at the first visit shows no significant abnormality. The likely explanation for this is a misdirected biopsy and a repeat colposcopy and biopsy is again advisable in 3 months.

LEARNING POINTS

1. The objectives of follow-up are to detect any residual or recurrent disease.
2. The success rate of treating CIN is between 90% and 95%.
3. Large lesions, high-grade lesions, incomplete excision, older patients and difficulties at the time of treatment are all risk factors predictive of treatment failure.
4. Most treatment failures are detected in the first 12 months following treatment.
5. Recurrence is more likely when a prolonged period of cytologically negative follow-up has been observed following initial treatment (about 2 years).
6. Follow-up is based on cytology. Additional colposcopy may enhance the early diagnosis of small residual lesions.

7. Invasive cancer occurs in about 1 in 1000 treated cases; microinvasion in about one in 1000 treated cases.
8. Patients with a current history of CIN treated by hysterectomy require cytological follow-up.

MCQS

33. After local ablative or excisional treatment of CIN:
    a. The risk of frank invasive cancer is 1 in 1000
    b. Most residual disease will be recognized within 12 months
    c. Colposcopy and cytology should be performed within 3 months
    d. Recurrent disease is more likely than residual disease
    e. A success rate of between 90% and 95% can be expected

34. Follow-up for treated CIN:
    a. Includes colposcopy at 12 months in all women
    b. Is more likely to be abnormal in women who have had high-grade lesions treated
    c. Is based on colposcopy rather than cytology
    d. May be normal despite the presence of residual disease
    e. Requires an annual smear for three years

35. After a hysterectomy:
    a. Women who have never had an abnormal smear require no further cytological surveillance
    b. Colposcopy and cytology should be performed at 6 weeks
    c. Colposcopy and cytology should be a part of follow-up if CIN is present
    d. There is a risk of VaIN in all patients
    e. Lugol's iodine is more reliable in detecting residual CIN than acetic acid

36. In untreated patients with abnormal smears:
    a. Colposcopy may be normal despite a moderately dyskaryotic smear
    b. The preferred treatment for persistent dyskaryosis is ablation
    c. Two consecutively negative smears are required prior to discharge back to routine recall
    d. Random punch biopsies should be performed if colposcopy is normal
    e. A normal punch biopsy means that the patient can be discharged to recall

<table>
<tr><td>

13

</td><td>

The management of early invasion and adenocarcinoma-*in-situ* (AIS)

</td></tr>
</table>

F. G. Lawton

INTRODUCTION

Invasive cervical cancer occurs when the basement membrane is breached by the neoplastic process. The original definition of 'microinvasive' carcinoma was proposed by Mestwerdt in 1947 as a cancer penetrating up to 5 mm into the cervical stroma, but the definition of a microinvasive lesion has ranged from as little as 1 mm to as great as 9 mm. The extent of the problem is underlined by the fact that over the years nearly 20 definitions of 'microinvasion' have been used.

The most recent FIGO classification in 1995 (see Appendix A) defines Stage la as 'invasive cancer identified only microscopically'. Two subdivisions are recognized: Stage la1 – 'measured invasion of stroma no greater than 3 mm in depth and no wider than 7 mm'; and stage la2: 'measured invasion of stroma greater than 3 mm and no greater than 5 mm in depth and no wider than 7 mm'. The depth of the invasion should be taken from the base of the epithelium, either surface or glandular, from which it originates. Lesions wider than 7 mm should be included in Stage Ib, even if the degree of invasion is minimal.

Handbook of Colposcopy, edited by David Luesley, Mahmood Shafi and Joe Jordan. Published in 1996 by Chapman & Hall, London. ISBN 0 412 71550 3

SQUAMOUS MICROINVASION

Microinvasion is defined in order to identify a group of patients who are at minimal risk of lymph node metastases and who may therefore be treated with less than radical therapy. Although depth of invasion is the traditional parameter to define invasion, other criteria may be useful in defining prognosis and therefore treatment.

Tumour area is already incorporated into the FIGO definition to distinguish Stage Ia2 and Stage Ib cancer and empirically a tumour volume of 500 mm^3 defines the upper limit of microinvasion. Although this definition is fine in theory, the technical difficulties in evaluating tumour volume should be emphasized. Few pathology laboratories have the expertise or the time to evaluate cone biopsy specimens in such rigorous detail.

The presence of tumour cells within capillary spaces in the cervical stroma, so-called lymph–vascular (LV) space involvement, is also cited by some as of prognostic significance, although this remains controversial. In addition, there is argument as to what constitutes a lymph–vascular space. The endothelial lining of very small vascular channels may not be readily apparent and invasion may therefore be difficult to quantify. In microinvasive disease there appears to be no correlation between tumour grade and depth of invasion.

Diagnosis and treatment

By definition, a preclinical malignant lesion will usually present as an abnormal smear. The colposcopic appearances of high-grade CIN and microinvasion can be similar but occult cancer may be suspected by the finding of a raised, acetowhite area with an irregular contour, over which are atypical vessels or a mosaic or punctate pattern (Chapter 8). The cervix may appear colposcopically normal, the lesion being present within the cervical canal. It must be emphasized, however, that often a microinvasive lesion is only discovered as a result of histological examination of a cervical biopsy.

When such a biopsy is reported, the next step in management is to determine the depth of invasion of the lesion either by formal cone biopsy (Fig. 13.1), or, a more recent development and still perhaps controversial in this context, by large loop excision of the transformation zone (LLETZ) (Fig. 13.2). In order to obtain a suitable-sized specimen the latter should be undertaken under general anaesthetic.

Invasion less than 1 mm

Patients with invasion less than 1 mm, so-called 'early stromal invasion', have essentially a 0% chance of pelvic node metastases. Consequently, curative surgery could consist of cone biopsy alone if the surgical margins of the cone specimen were found to be free of disease. Simple hysterectomy is another

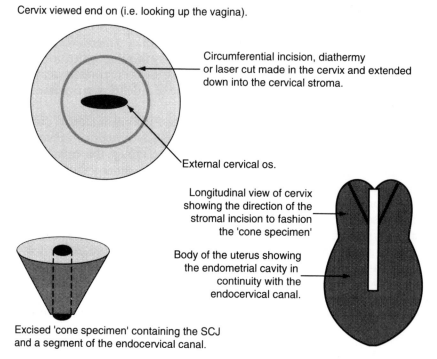

Cervix viewed end on (i.e. looking up the vagina).

Circumferential incision, diathermy or laser cut made in the cervix and extended down into the cervical stroma.

External cervical os.

Longitudinal view of cervix showing the direction of the stromal incision to fashion the 'cone specimen'

Body of the uterus showing the endometrial cavity in continuity with the endocervical canal.

Excised 'cone specimen' containing the SCJ and a segment of the endocervical canal.

Fig. 13.1 Diagrammatic representation of a cone biopsy of the cervix.

option, particularly if preservation of fertility is not an issue. A patient whose cone biopsy shows positive margins should be treated by simple hysterectomy or, rarely, by a further cone biopsy.

Invasion between 1 mm and 3 mm

Patients with microinvasion between 1 and 3 mm still have a less than 1% chance of nodal disease. It has been postulated that the risk of nodal disease increases after 3 mm invasion because LV channels are extremely narrow this close to the basement membrane and may not be able to accommodate and disseminate tumour cells. Therapeutic cone biopsy is adequate treatment for this group of patients if fertility is to be preserved; otherwise simple hysterectomy should be performed. Controversy exists as to whether such patients with evidence of LV space involvement could still be treated with simple surgery or whether pelvic lymph node dissection should be considered.

Invasion between 3 mm and 5 mm

Invasion between 3 mm and 5 mm carries a 5–8% risk of pelvic node disease and here some authors have advocated more radical surgery, particularly

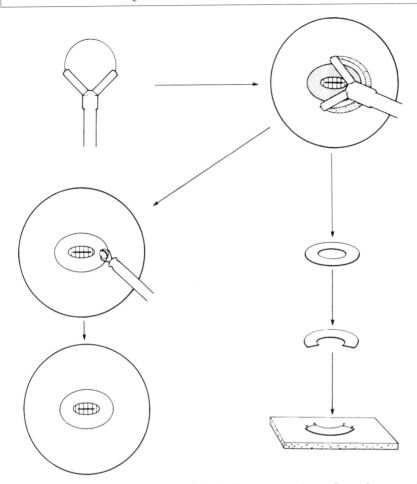

Fig. 13.2 LLETZ excision of a small, fully visible ectocervical transformation zone. A medium (white) loop is used for the procedure.

when the lesion is greater than 1 cm in diameter, or 500 mm^3 in volume, or shows the presence of LV space invasion. In such a case a so-called modified radical or 'type II' hysterectomy (a type III hysterectomy is the standard radical hysterectomy), originally described by Wertheim, which excises the medial portion of the cardinal ligaments and the uterosacral ligaments, might be recommended. A limited pelvic lymphadenectomy or removal of clinically enlarged pelvic nodes might also be carried out. No vaginal cuff need be taken except in rare cases where there is colposcopic evidence of spread of disease to the vault.

No data from randomized studies to assess how radical surgery should be in these cases are available but it should be emphasized that deaths from invasive cervical cancer after conservative surgery for microinvasive disease are extremely rare. The 30-year experience of the Norwegian Radium Hospital suggests that only about 2% of patients treated within this type of protocol will die of recurrent cervical cancer. These variations in management are a consequence of our shortcomings in understanding the natural history of microinvasive cervical cancer and concerns regarding, on the one hand, possible undertreatment of node positive disease and, on the other, the morbidity associated with radical pelvic surgery.

ADENOCARCINOMA-*IN-SITU* (AIS)

Invasive cervical cancers containing glandular elements comprise 20% of cases, a number which has increased some fourfold in the last 25 years. It is generally believed that AIS is the precursor lesion in adenocarcinoma but it is interesting to note that the *in-situ* lesion seems to be detected much less commonly than its invasive counterpart, a very different picture from the equivalent squamous neoplasms. This probably reflects changes in the location of the transformation zone – its upper limit moves into the endocervical canal as a woman becomes older and the mean age of women with AIS in some series is around 40 years – and the fact that AIS cells may be mistaken for normal endocervical cells.

Adenocarcinoma-*in-situ* is a more difficult pathological entity to define than its squamous counterpart. The earliest atypical nuclear patterns are subtle and may be confused with microglandular hyperplasia. In addition, once the gland has been invaded, penetration of the adjacent basement membrane cannot be measured with any accuracy. Thus the lesion is either AIS or invasive adenocarcinoma; the term 'microinvasion' should not be used.

The majority of cases of AIS are identified in cervical biopsies or cones obtained in the management of squamous lesions or in uterine specimens removed for other pathologies. In addition, abnormal glandular cells may be detected on a cervical smear. Over 60% of cases of AIS coincide with CIN or microinvasive disease. The two separate *in-situ* lesions often merge in the transformation zone, but occasionally squamous and glandular elements are mixed together as an adenosquamous carcinoma-*in-situ*.

Diagnosis and management

Although abnormal glandular cells may be found on a smear, no dedicated screening test exists. The situation may change with the use of a Cytobrush in conjunction with an Ayre's spatula. In addition, there are no diagnostic colposcopic appearances and this, coupled with the fact that the lesions are often small and out of sight up the endocervical canal, means that the role of colposcopically directed biopsies is limited. The only way to obtain an accurate histological diagnosis and to determine the extent of the lesion is to carry out a cone biopsy. Controversy exists as to whether this can be considered a therapeutic as well as a diagnostic procedure. The potential role for LLETZ excision of these lesions has not been explored, but it is likely that the size of the excision biopsy achievable by LLETZ would preclude adequate sampling of the endocervical canal and it is therefore not currently recommended.

Some authors consider, since the abnormality may occur anywhere in the endocervical canal and a high lesion may not be excised by cone biopsy, that only hysterectomy can ensure complete removal of the entire cervical canal and can thus be considered definitive therapy. Vaginal hysterectomy has obvious advantages over the abdominal route. The ovaries can be conserved. Others cite studies, where cone biopsy has been followed by hysterectomy, that have shown in general that if the cone margins are free of disease, then the hysterectomy specimen will also be negative. Microcolpohysteroscopy may have a role in defining the upper end of the lesion, so tailoring the size of the cone to the extent of the abnormality.

Follow-up for patients treated by cone biopsy is problematical and great care must be taken to adequately sample the residual endocervical canal, which may be scarred considerably. The use of a Cytobrush or endocervical curette may facilitate sampling. It should be emphasized that one study concluded that 'since one cannot expect to be able to thoroughly assess the endocervix over time, conservative management is dangerous....'

SUMMARY

Definitive therapy for AIS remains undetermined. In selected cases cone biopsy seems curative but it should be remembered that follow-up in most studies is short . There has been a report of recurrent AIS within 13 months of cone biopsy and another of a patient who died of invasive adenocarcinoma 16 years after hysterectomy for AIS.

LEARNING POINTS

1. FIGO criteria used to define microinvasive cervical cancer include depth of invasion below the basement membrane and surface area of the tumour.
2. Controversial prognostic factors include tumour volume and the presence of lymph–vascular space involvement.
3. With a depth of invasion of 1 mm or less (early stromal invasion), the chance of lymph node metastases is essentially zero and cone biopsy is a curative procedure.
4. With 1–3 mm invasion nodal disease occurs in less than 1% of cases. If fertility is to be preserved, cone biopsy is curative, otherwise hysterectomy is recommended.

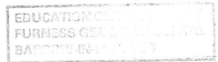
EDUCATION
FURNESS GEN
BA

5. The chance of nodal disease with invasion of 3–5 mm is 5–8%.
6. The incidence of adenocarcinoma of the cervix has increased over the last two decades.
7. There is no glandular equivalent of microinvasive squamous cell cancer: the lesion is either '*in-situ*' or invasive.
8. Cone biopsy may be considered curative for AIS, but a lesion high in the cervical canal may be missed by the procedure. The only way to remove the entire canal is by hysterectomy.

MCQS

37. Microinvasive cervical carcinoma:
   a. May be defined as a lesion visible on the cervix to the naked eye with a depth of invasion of 2 mm
   b. May be cured by LLETZ
   c. Carries a risk of nodal metastases of around 1%
   d. May be defined as a lesion invading 3 mm or less below the basement membrane

38. Adenocarcinoma of the cervix:
   a. Is increasing in incidence
   b. Microinvasion is defined in terms of depth of invasion into the stroma from the nearest gland
   c. Over 60% of cases of AIS coincide with in-situ or microinvasive squamous lesions
   d. AIS treated by hysterectomy should include bilateral oophorectomy

39. Pelvic lymphadenectomy should be considered:
   a. In cases of adenosquamous carcinoma-*in-situ*
   b. In microinvasive cervical cancer with LVS invasion
   c. For a lesion with a volume greater than 500 mm^3
   d. For a lesion invading 3 mm below the basement membrane

40. Fertility may be conserved:
   a. With a microinvasive lesion 1–3 mm below the basement membrane
   b. With a Stage Ia2 lesion
   c. In a case of AIS
   d. In a case of a mixed AIS/CIN lesion

41. Cone biopsy alone can be considered curative in cases where:
   a. The depth of invasion is greater than 5 mm
   b. The surface area of the lesion is greater than 50 mm^2
   c. The volume of the lesion is greater than 500 mm^3
   d. There is adenocarcinoma-*in-situ*

Human papillomavirus: its role in aetiology and screening

14

G. P. Downey

INTRODUCTION

Despite an extensive cervical screening programme there has as yet been little decrease in the incidence of cervical cancer in the United Kingdom. The reasons for this are manifold and include poor technique in sampling, failure to target the 'at risk' population and deficiency in the sensitivity of cytology. Cytology is a rather inexact science relying on exfoliated cells to give information on the underlying cervical epithelium. Although the test is specific for cervical intraepithelial neoplasia, with a low false-positive rate, there is a well recognized deficiency in sensitivity, the latter known to be proportional to the lesion size. Up to 30% of tests are falsely negative (range 6–30%), while 30% of cervical cancers are associated with a (apparently) normal cervical smear within 3 years of diagnosis. We also know that between 16% and 30% of women with a mildly dyskaryotic smear have in fact high-grade cervical disease on colposcopy and biopsy; thus the ideal management of such women is immediate referral to colposcopy. However, this would overwhelm an already taxed colposcopy service and inevitably lead to overtreatment of some women if a 'see and treat' policy were employed. The consequence of these factors is the search for a reliable alternative or secondary screening procedure

Handbook of Colposcopy, edited by David Luesley, Mahmood Shafi and Joe Jordan. Published in 1996 by Chapman & Hall, London. ISBN 0 412 71550 3

which will help identify those women requiring immediate referral to colposcopy and rationalization of resources.

HUMAN PAPILLOMAVIRUS

That Human papillomavirus (HPV) was important in the aetiology of CIN and cervical cancer was first proposed by zur Hausen in 1984. Since then there has been a wealth of epidemiological and compelling scientific evidence to substantiate this claim. Initial studies were methodologically flawed as they relied on cytology to diagnose and follow up CIN; thus the underlying histology was not reliably established. Combined with this were the use of different tests for HPV with varying sensitivities and specificities, and a lack of knowledge and understanding of the natural history of a disease often distorted by treatment. Despite these difficulties a large volume of epidemiological and molecular biological evidence has accumulated which now makes it virtually certain that specific HPV types are the main cause of most cases of CIN and cervical cancer.

One of the problems of ascribing the virus an aetiological role in the development of CIN was its high prevalence in the normal population, initial poorly controlled studies finding erroneously that the virus was almost ubiquitous. However, this was later found to be the result of contamination of the HPV assay used. The recent case-control studies find that approximately 10% of normal women will test positive for oncogenic HPV DNAs, and 85–90% of women with a high-grade lesion will test positive. The different viral types found in the lower genital tract have been subdivided into 'low' and 'high' risk groups in that they tend to be associated with, but are not exclusive to, low-grade and high-grade lesions. By far the most important high-risk type in the UK is HPV 16, which accounts for 60–85% of high-grade CIN and cervical cancer, with HPV types 18, 31 and 33 accounting for most of the rest. The virus is transmitted by sexual intercourse; infection is often transient and can cause mild, reversible cytological changes, although in a minority of women infection persists and results in cervical disease (Table 14.1).

HUMAN PAPILLOMAVIRUS BIOLOGY

The viruses are a family of double-stranded DNA viruses. The viral genome is divided into functional gene regions: 'early' (E) and 'late' (L) regions. The early

Table 14.1 The HPV subtypes in relation to the oncogenic risk

Low-risk	6	11	42	43	44						
High-risk	16	18	31	33	35	39	45	51	52	56	58

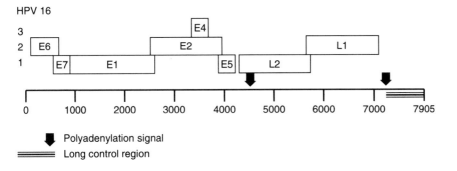

Fig. 14.1 Diagrammatic representation of the HPV 16 genome showing the early (E) and late (L) open reading frames.

regions contain eight open reading frames (ORFs) coding proteins in viral maintenance and replication while the two late region ORFs produce proteins that form the viral capsid and are termed structural proteins (Fig. 14.1).

Transfection of human keratinocytes with Human papillomavirus causes cellular transformation, immortalization and integration of the virus into host cell DNA when the cells progress to a more oncogenic phenotype with each cell division typical of cervical intraepithelial cells. The viral integration appears to play an important role in the oncogenic process as the genes that control cell growth remain intact following integration while other viral genes are lost. The important genes are E6 and E7, which have been found to form complexes with the tumour suppressor genes p53 and p105 RB with a subsequent loss of control of cell growth. It is only recently that the well controlled clinical studies have been performed that substantiate the laboratory findings.

DIAGNOSIS OF HUMAN PAPILLOMAVIRUS INFECTION

HPV is tropic for epithelium and will only replicate in terminally differentiated keratinocytes, so there is no culture medium for analysis. Serological tests are unreliable and detection therefore depends on DNA hybridization techniques. Probes for the detection of HPV have been present from the early 1980s and from a research perspective this molecular technology has yielded enormous benefits.

Southern blot

Southern blot was regarded as the 'gold standard' test for identifying HPV infection. Essentially, the cellular DNA is extracted from cells and biopsy material by SDS proteinase K digestion and purified with a phenol/chloroform mix. The sample is then digested with various restriction enzymes and the resulting fragments are separated according to size by electrophoresis on an agarose gel. The various HPV types are labelled with radioactive probes and hybridization on to a nitrocellulose filter allows their identification. Southern blot can detect 0.01–0.1 copies of viral DNA per cell. While the test can be highly sensitive and specific it requires a large amount of DNA, is time-consuming and loses sensitivity when applied to cervical cytology specimens, and is thus not suitable for mass screening.

Dot blot

This technique is similar to Southern blot in that it uses the same DNA extraction technique; once extracted the DNA is not digested but applied directly on to a filter after denaturation. The sensitivity of the test is lower but larger numbers can be assessed more rapidly. Highly stringent conditions are required to prevent false-positive results.

Filter *in situ* hybridization

Cells are filtered directly on to a membrane where they are lysed and denatured in alkaline buffer. The DNA is neutralized and the membrane is baked for 4 hours at 80°C. Hybridization with cloned specific probes is then performed under high stringency conditions to ensure specific recognition between the probe and target. The membrane is then washed and processed for auto-radiography. The rapidity of results is paid for by a low sensitivity, biopsy samples being required to ensure enough DNA is available, and the technique is thus is not suitable for mass screening.

In situ hybridization

This allows direct visualization of HPV DNA or RNA in cytological preparations or tissue sections from frozen or fresh specimens. The main benefit of this technique is that it can be applied to archival material which is paraffin-embedded. The sample is treated with proteinase K, denatured and then hybridized with labelled DNA or RNA probes. The samples are then washed and prepared for autoradiography. The technique is technically demanding and of varying sensitivity, depending on whether a radioactive or biotin-labelled probe is used.

The polymerase chain reaction

The polymerase chain reaction (PCR) allows for the enzymatic synthesis of millions of copies of a segment of target DNA. A pair of short DNA fragments known as primers is synthesized to be complementary to sequences on opposite strands of DNA flanking the fragment to be amplified. The DNA sample is denatured and the primers anneal to each of the single strands. The annealed primers then extend towards each other from the 3′ hydroxyl ends by a DNA polymerase in the presence of a mixture of deoxynucleotide triphosphates (dNTPs), using the target sequence as a template. This initial extension then provides the template for subsequent replication and so the original sequence is amplified exponentially. The amplified product is then detected by ultraviolet light on an ethidium-bromide-treated agarose gel which has been electrophoresed. This technique is exquisitely sensitive, requiring only one copy of HPV per 10^5–10^6 cells. It is a useful tool for research purposes and as such is now taken as the new 'gold standard' but, because of its very high sensitivity and vulnerability to contamination, leading to false-positive results, it is not useful in mass screening.

Solution hybridization or hybrid capture

This is one of the oldest nucleic acid hybridization techniques. More recently the technique has been refined to be more sensitive and specific than filter hybridization yet still simple to perform. A commercial form of the solution known as hybrid capture is a simple, non-radioactive immunoassay that employs RNA probes to detect single-stranded target DNA. Hybrids are captured on to the surface of a plastic tube by immobilized antibodies specific for RNA–DNA hybrids. The unreacted RNA probe is not immobilized to the tube surface and is eliminated by washing. Detection of the positive specimens is achieved by reacting the hybrids with an alkaline-phosphatase-conjugated RNA–DNA antibody, followed by incubation in a chemiluminescent substrate (Lumiphos). Alkaline phosphate cleaves the Lumiphos, resulting in emission of light in direct proportion to the quantity of captured hybrid. This technique can detect up to 16 types of HPV in a single reaction. Initial trials reveal a high sensitivity and specificity for all clinically relevant HPV infection and it is believed to be the technique of choice for mass screening.

SCREENING

HPV screening in the primary setting

In initial studies the value of HPV 16 only was assessed to determine if it was useful to detect high-grade disease in an asymptomatic general practice population. However, the prevalence of infection in the normal population was high (16%) and the HPV 16 assay, assessed in a qualitative manner, was no better than cervical cytology in the detection of cervical disease; however, a combination of the two was better than either alone. More recently, Cuzick *et al.* included HPV types 18, 31 and 33 in the semiquantitative assay and found that in almost 2000 asymptomatic women with no previous history of cervical disease the combination of HPV testing with cervical cytology was useful in the detection of those women with cervical intraepithelial neoplasia and had a greater sensitivity than either test alone. A much larger multicentre study is proposed prior to the proposed introduction of the test to the national screening programme.

HPV screening and mild dyskaryosis

By far the greatest problem facing the clinician is the 250 000 women with a mildly dyskaryotic smear report. As there is a recognized undercall rate of up to 30%, early referral to colposcopy would be the ideal management. However, resources are limited and this ideal is not practicable. The effect of the introduction of a semiquantitative PCR assay in determining which women with a mildly dyskaryotic smear report have in fact high-grade disease has been formally assessed in a study by Bavin *et al.* and confirmed by Cuzick and his colleagues. Each patient had a repeat smear, colposcopy and directed biopsy and a HPV 16 semiquantitative assay. HPV 16 alone was no better than cervical cytology but a combination of the two improved the sensitivity of screening without diminishing the specificity. A strong association was found in all these studies with medium/high copy numbers of HPV 16 and high-grade cervical disease irrespective of the degree of dyskaryosis on cytology. Once again the introduction of other HPV (types 18, 31, 33 and 35) has improved the detection rate of CIN 3 to 84%. Numerous groups are attempting to improve the sensitivity by using different types of HPV primer, i.e. type-specific rather than consensus or a combination of the two, but the results to date are disappointing.

HPV screening in moderate to severe dyskaryosis

Patients who have moderate to severely dyskaryotic smears will be referred for colposcopy regardless of their HPV status as these cytological results are much more sensitive and specific for high-grade disease than minor cytological abnormalities. Therefore the introduction of a HPV test would not influence clinical care but is of interest in a research setting.

LEARNING POINTS

1. The present cervical screening programme has recognized deficiencies in sensitivity with false-negative results and undercall of high-grade lesions. Therefore secondary screening measures which are sensitive, specific, acceptable to the patient and cost-effective have been proposed.

2. Human papillomavirus is a DNA virus sexually transmitted to the lower genital tract whose natural history closely mimics that of cervical intra-epithelial neoplasia. There is a wealth of epidemiological evidence supporting an aetiological role of the virus in both CIN and cervical cancer. These findings have been supported by compelling experimental evidence confirming both a transforming and an immortalizing effect of the virus on human keratinocytes.

3. There is no culture medium for Human papillomavirus and detection relies on hybridization techniques. Of the numerous techniques available the polymerase chain reaction (PCR) is by far the most sensitive and is useful for research purposes. Hybrid capture is the most reliable and sensitive technique to use in the detection of all clinically relevant HPV infection.

4. There are numerous viral subtypes, only a few of which are related to the lower genital tract. These are classified into 'low' and 'high' risk types because of their association with low-grade and high-grade disease. The main high-risk types are 16 and 18, with 31 and 33 playing an important minor role.

5. HPV assay alone, whether assessed in a qualitative or semiquantitative manner, is inadequate to reliably detect high-grade cervical disease, albeit in a primary care setting or in assessment of women referred with a mildly dyskaryotic smear report. However, a combination of HPV 16, 18, 31 and 33 assay assessed in a semiquantitative manner with conventional cervical cytology can improve the detection of high-grade disease. Employing such a combined strategy may help rationalize colposcopy resources and target referral to those who require colposcopic assessment most.

MCQS

42. The following criteria are met by HPV screening:
    a. It is highly sensitive for all grades of cervical disease when performed in a qualitative manner
    b. The polymerase chain reaction is the most useful test in mass screening
    c. Medium/high copy numbers of HPV 16 can predict high-grade cervical disease more accurately than cervical cytology
    d. When assessed in a semiquantitative manner, HPV screening may replace conventional cytology
    e. HPV types 16, 18, 31 and 33 are the most useful types to screen for in the UK

15 Difficult situations and management problems

D. M. Luesley

ABNORMAL SMEARS IN PREGNANCY

There are two ways in which pregnant women present with abnormal smears. They may have a smear taken during the pregnancy or they may have had an abnormal smear and become pregnant before investigation and or treatment. Regarding the former, there is really no justification to take an *ad hoc* smear during pregnancy unless there is a clinical indication. In some situations it might be the only opportunity of taking a smear and this might be a justification. The quality of smears taken in pregnancy and indeed the early puerperium (6 weeks) is generally poorer and the risk of false negatives is higher.

Abnormal smear recognized for the first time in pregnancy

The recommendations for referral for colposcopy are the same in pregnancy as in the non-pregnant state. Current UK recommendations are that all smears reported as moderately dyskaryotic or worse should be colposcoped. Lesser abnormalities should have a repeat smear 6 months following the first abnormality and should be referred if still abnormal. There is an argument for altering these recommendations based on recently published data and one might also consider the possibility of undercall or sampling error, both likely to be increased in pregnancy as a result of poor-quality smears and the much larger transformation zone that is a characteristic of the pregnant cervix.

Handbook of Colposcopy, edited by David Luesley, Mahmood Shafi and Joe Jordan. Published in 1996 by Chapman & Hall, London. ISBN 0 412 71550 3

For these reasons, and of course the more highly charged emotional state that prevails in this situation, colposcopy for all but borderline changes is perhaps the best option. As more women enter the screening programme the need for *ad hoc* pregnancy smears has declined and therefore the number of abnormal smear cases identified in pregnancy is also less. This means that an immediate referral policy will not significantly alter the workload of the colposcopy service.

Colposcopy in pregnancy

The procedure is no different from that performed in the non-pregnant state. Much more reassurance is required, with emphasis on the fact that the procedure will not harm the fetus or cause miscarriage. The cervix changes as pregnancy advances, colposcopy becoming progressively more difficult. Because of this, misinterpretation is possible even in experienced hands. Women rarely need colposcopy in the third trimester, perhaps the only exception being late booking and a clinically suspicious cervix.

The major changes that affect colposcopy are as follows.

1. The cervix is larger.
2. Access can be more difficult.
3. The transformation zone is larger.
4. There is more mucus and it is more tenacious.
5. There is much more metaplasia
6. The cervix is softer and much more vascular (biopsy may be more morbid and small biopsies may be more easily damaged).

It is essential to take time to visualize the whole transformation zone carefully as a small field of CIN may be present within much wider areas of metaplasia. While accurate grading of CIN is important, there is a tendency to overdiagnose in pregnancy. This may reflect the increased vascularity of the cervix.

The woman will need a large cervical biopsy if there is any suspicion of an invasive process based on the smear or on colposcopy. This is the most reliable way of excluding invasion. Small targeted biopsies are not ideal to exclude invasion. As treatment of CIN is rarely if ever indicated during pregnancy there is little justification for taking directed biopsies. The reasons for this are the following.

1. They are unreliable in the diagnosis of invasive disease.
2. In pregnancy there is more chance of an unsatisfactory sample.
3. In pregnancy there is an increased risk of haemorrhage.

For these reasons, large biopsies are preferable and are only performed if colposcopy and/or cytology suggests the possibility of invasion. Our own clinic protocol incorporates these ideas in a relatively simple structure that allows for minimal intervention in women with preinvasive disease yet early diagnosis of those with invasion.

Abnormal smears in pregnancy: a protocol for management

1. **Any abnormal smear other than borderline:** Colposcopy within 4 weeks.
2. **Colposcopy and cytology suggest no more than CIN 1:** Repeat assessment 3 months after delivery.
3. **Colposcopy and cytology suggest CIN 2 or 3:** Repeat assessment at end of second trimester.
4. **Colposcopy and or cytology suggest invasion:** Wedge biopsy under general anaesthetic.

Postpartum assessments

These do not differ from those in the normal non-pregnant population. Occasionally the vagina and cervix appear relatively hypo-oestrogenic, particularly in breast-feeding mothers. If this significantly hinders colposcopy and cytology, a 6-week course of local oestrogen often improves matters.

Abnormal smear prior to a pregnancy

Women who have had adequately treated CIN do not require any additional surveillance during pregnancy. If a follow-up smear is required, this should be deferred until at least 3 months following delivery. The only group who should be offered colposcopy are those who have not had a negative smear after treatment where there are grounds to suspect incomplete removal of CIN, i.e. after incomplete loop excision of large lesions.

Women who have an abnormal smear but have not yet been investigated are managed as for those whose first smear was taken during pregnancy.

Women who have had CIN 1 (or less) diagnosed should be reassessed 3 months following delivery. Women who have had high-grade disease (CIN 2 and CIN 3) diagnosed should be reassessed 6 months following the diagnosis and only rebiopsied (large biopsy) if it is felt that there may have been progression to invasion. Standard approaches are used to treat high-grade disease 3 months postpartum.

There are no published data supporting the concept of more rapid progression of CIN to invasion in pregnancy.

POSTMENOPAUSAL SMEARS

Women over the age of 65 years who have had regular and normal screening are at very little risk of developing cervical cancer. The screening programme therefore stops at this age. However, cancer of the cervix is still more prevalent in older women and screening is maintained well into the menopause.

As a result of oestrogen loss profound changes affect the genital tract, including the cervix. There is an overall shrinkage of the tissues with an inversion of the cervix and as a consequence the squamocolumnar junction may appear to recede up the endocervical canal. Along with these changes the epithelium becomes thinner and more easily traumatized, there is less glycogenation of squamous cells and the pH of the vagina increases, removing one level of vaginal defence. Smears from postmenopausal women therefore contain fewer cells and less mature squames and are less likely to adequately sample the squamo-columnar junction. In postmenopausal women there is a greater incidence of unsatisfactory smear reports. There would seem to be good theoretical grounds for providing oestrogen replacement in such women and then repeating the smear. However, no published data support this clinical practice.

Colposcopy in the menopausal woman

Colposcopy is also less reliable in menopausal women. It is more difficult to fully visualize the squamocolumnar junction and more likely to traumatize the ectocervix. Biopsies, which should always include the SCJ, will nearly always require some type of conization. This is because the shrinkage and inversion of the cervix cause the squamocolumnar junction to recede into the endo-cervical canal.

Major degrees of cytological abnormality in elderly women should always raise the possibility of invasive disease – usually cervical, but occasionally even endometrial cancer might present because of abnormalities on a smear. Such smear results must be thoroughly investigated, with early recourse to a large biopsy and endometrial assessment. As future fertility is not an issue in these women fear of anatomical distortion of the residual cervix should not deter the clinician from acquiring large biopsies.

The indications for colposcopy are the same as in the premenopausal state. There is however a greater need for assessment if cervical smears are repeatedly unsatisfactory. Just as cytology is more likely to be unsatisfactory, so is colposcopy. Apart from an increased chance of not visualizing the SCJ, the atrophic appearances can result in unusual vessel patterns. Prior cytology can easily strip the thinned epithelium, leaving exposed stroma. In this situation the colposcopist cannot be sure that the removed epithelium was normal. The reaction to iodine is often incomplete because of poor glycogenation and that to acetic acid may be false-positive because of stripping.

In situations where the smear definitely confirms dyskaryosis, conization is required unless colposcopy is absolutely satisfactory. If the smear shows very minor or borderline changes, treatment with oestrogen (locally or parent-erally) followed by repeat cytology and colposcopy after 3 months is the preferred course of action.

ABNORMAL VAGINAL VAULT SMEARS

Women who have had a hysterectomy with CIN present require vaginal vault smears for follow-up. Other hysterectomized women do not. *De novo* vaginal intraepithelial neoplasia (VaIN) is so rare as not to warrant a screening test. Very occasionally women will have an abnormal smear who have not previously had CIN. In most of these the cause is HPV only.

The vast majority of women who have an abnormal vaginal vault smear will have a history of CIN. To keep the number of these cases to a minimum all women undergoing hysterectomy should have an up-to-date cervical smear and colposcopy, if this is abnormal, before hysterectomy. Colposcopy serves two functions in this situation. First, it helps to exclude the presence of invasive disease, for which simple hysterectomy would be inappropriate. Second, the colposcopist can see if there is any vaginal extension of CIN. If there is any evidence of vaginal extension, removing an appropriate cuff of vaginal tissue at the time of hysterectomy (vaginal or abdominal) should ensure complete excision of any intraepithelial disease. A careful histopathological assessment of the vaginal margins will determine whether excision is complete. Excision status determines the follow-up strategy.

1. **CIN is confirmed in the hysterectomy specimen and is completely excised:** In this situation perform a repeat vault smear 6 and 18 months after the hysterectomy. Discontinue follow-up if both are negative.
2. **CIN is confirmed and excision is either uncertain or incomplete:** Follow-up is as for any treated patient with CIN. Perform vault smears 6 and 12 months posthysterectomy and annually thereafter to 5 years. If all the follow-up smears are negative 3-yearly recall suffices.

Any abnormal vault smear requires a colposcopic assessment.

Vaginal vault colposcopy

This is more difficult than standard colposcopy. First, there is no transformation zone and second, scarring and distortion of the vault because of posthysterectomy healing can make full visualization of the suture line difficult. This is particularly so at the angles, where, depending upon the technique of vaginal vault closure employed, deep inaccessible pockets can form. If these are present it is important to try and evert them with the aid of a small skin hook.

If abnormal epithelium is present it shares the same appearances as intraepithelial neoplasia with an intact cervix such as punctomosaic vascular pattern and acetowhitening. Any atypical areas should be biopsied. This is also more problematic. Areas isolated from the suture line can be biopsied in outpatients but the standard punch biopsy forceps may be difficult to use or cause an excessive crush artefact as there is no subepithelial stroma. Atypical areas at or on the vault scar pose an even more difficult problem as sequestration of intraepithelial disease beneath the suture line often occurs. Some have suggested leaving the vaginal vault open after hysterectomy in all cases of intraepithelial neoplasia, to reduce the chance of burying CIN. This method of closure seems theoretically sound but has not been proven.

To cut a good biopsy from the non-scarred part of the vagina use a long-handled Keyes punch. A formal knife excisional biopsy is the best technique when the atypical epithelium involves the angles or suture line. If excisional biopsy confirms VaIN and complete excision, the patient is followed up as for after TAH. If incomplete excision is confirmed we tend to observe only those whose original and recurrent disease was low-grade, but perform a formal upper vaginectomy in confirmed high-grade disease. This is because several small series on posthysterectomy VaIN have suggested a relatively high prevalence of carcinoma.

An alternative to upper vaginectomy is vaginal vault irradiation. This can be difficult to administer, has the potential to result in sexual morbidity and may also make subsequent interpretation of vaginal vault smears difficult.

CERVICAL STENOSIS

Stenosis is a term usually reserved for situations in which narrowing of a structure causes abnormal function. Stenosis of the endocervical canal can cause symptoms such as dysmenorrhoea and might also result in problems with conceiving or labour.

Stenosis can also cause the squamocolumnar junction to become hidden within the canal resulting in non-representative smears and unsatisfactory colposcopy. Treatment of CIN is one of the most common causes of cervical stenosis. It occurs in up to 20% of cases managed by formal cold knife conization but usually in 2% or less of cases managed by local destruction or local excision. It occurs most frequently in women who are amenorrhoeic after cervical surgery (i.e. menopausal women). Reducing the length of canal removed reduces the risk of stenosis.

Women who are symptomatic require treatment. Cervical dilatation and/or recanalization by laser can be attempted but this usually only provides short term relief. Many symptomatic women will eventually need a hysterectomy.

Treatment is not usually required in asymptomatic women unless:

1. **High-grade disease was present and was incompletely excised:** In this situation there is no reliable method of follow-up. Older women or women who have completed their families should consider hysterectomy in this situation.
2. **Pelvic examination suggests uterine enlargement:** The possibility of either a haematometra or a pyometra should be considered. There is an

increased risk of endometrial pathology in these situations and again satisfactory surveillance or investigation is not possible. Hysterectomy should be considered.

3. **Either situation 1 or 2 prevails but hysterectomy is not an option:** The canal should be dilated or vaporized at least to allow endocervical and or endometrial tissue to be biopsied. Women should be counselled that such measures are usually temporary and that re-stenosis is possible. In selected cases, an endocervical stent can be placed after dilatation. This prolongs the time before which further dilatation is required and may allow enough time for conception, should this be desired.

LEARNING POINTS

1. Pregnancy and the puerperium are not ideal times to take a cervical smear. The quality of the smear can be affected by the pregnant or puerperal state.
2. There is no indication to treat CIN in pregnancy.
3. The main reason for taking a biopsy in pregnancy is to exclude invasion. A large biopsy is required to achieve this reliably.
4. The natural history of CIN is not believed to be affected by pregnancy.
5. The physiological changes associated with the menopause make cytology and colposcopy more difficult.
6. As invasive disease is more common in postmenopausal women, there should be early recourse to excisional biopsies such as a cone biopsy.
7. Oestrogen replacement may be valuable in improving both cytology and colposcopy in postmenopausal women.
8. Cone biopsy is the most common cause of cervical stenosis.
9. Cervical stenosis can cause symptoms and make cytology and colposcopy unreliable.
10. All women having a hysterectomy should have evidence of a recent cervical smear.
11. All women with abnormal cervical smears should be colposcoped prior to hysterectomy.

MCQS

43. During pregnancy
    a. CIN is more likely to progress to cancer
    b. The transformation zone becomes smaller
    c. CIN should be treated by laser
    d. Wedge biopsy is the preferred method of excluding invasion
    e. The endocervical speculum should not be used

Colposcopy in the setting of a genitourinary clinic | 16

D. A. Hicks

SOME STATISTICS

Around 300 000 women are seen annually in the Genitourinary Medicine (GUM) clinics of the UK as new patients. Cervical smears taken from these patients account for around 2% of the 4.5 million smears taken nationally each year.

90 GUM clinics perform colposcopy, and three-quarters of these treat cervical intraepithelial neoplasia (CIN), with one-quarter referring patients on to their gynaecological colleagues. Colposcopy tends to be performed only on existing clinic patients, since direct referral from general practice is unusual.

Around 10 500 new patients are seen *per annum* in GUM colposcopy clinics, with the colposcope used in some GUM clinics to visualize other parts of the male and female lower genital and anal tracts.

ARE GUM PATIENTS A HIGH-RISK GROUP FOR CIN AND/OR CERVICAL CANCER?

Consider some of the suggested risk factors for squamous carcinoma of the cervix. These are:

1. Early coital debut
2. Multiple sexual partners
3. Smoking

Handbook of Colposcopy, edited by David Luesley, Mahmood Shafi and Joe Jordan. Published in 1996 by Chapman & Hall, London. ISBN 0 412 71550 3

4. Human papillomavirus
5. Immunosuppression
6. Suggested infective agents:
   a. Herpes simplex virus
   b. Epstein–Barr virus
   c. *Trichomonas vaginalis*
   d. *Chlamydia trachomatis*
7. Lack of participation in the cytology screening system.

The female GUM population generally could be considered therefore to constitute a high-risk population. The idea of being able to identify such a population in order to target resources is attractive.

Most of these factors, however, carry only relatively weak associations with risk, and it is currently impossible to identify the population which, if targeted within the programme, would substantially alter its success.

Remember also that the majority of women attending GUM clinics are under the age of 25 years. This age group contributes less than 2% of all cases of invasive cervical carcinoma and only 0.1% of the total deaths from this cause. It is women over 45 years of age who make up 63% of new cases of invasive carcinoma and 82% of deaths.

Since it is more accurately a short lapse of time between menarche and coital debut, rather than absolute age at first sexual intercourse, that confers risk, it is not appropriate to perform cervical cytology on teenage women simply because they have been sexually active for any particular number of years. The incidence of cervical carcinoma in teenagers is only 2 per million.

Similarly, women with a history of genital Human papillomavirus (HPV) or Herpes simplex virus (HSV) infection have not yet been shown to benefit from more regular screening than National Programme intervals. Even if we assume that viruses pose a risk for the development of squamous carcinoma subsequently, it may be many years after infection. The woman may therefore be possibly disadvantaged in experiencing 'smear fatigue' when her initial smears are normal, with the system having to bear the cost of the increased number of smears.

The greatest contribution to the screening system for GUM clinics must therefore be 'opportunistic' cervical cytology, i.e. smearing women who through, for example the lack of a general practitioner or fixed address, have not been recognized, or invited by the computer database, and also those who have not had a cervical smear taken within the previous 5 years (the time period recommended in nationally agreed guidelines).

INFECTIONS, CYTOLOGY AND COLPOSCOPY

It is possible that an 'inflammatory smear' report may indicate the presence of an infective process (Plate 9). Specific organisms which may be identified

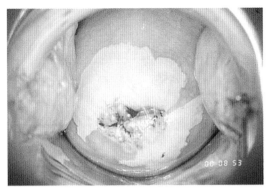

Plate 1 The atypical transformation zone: an extreme example of acetowhite change.

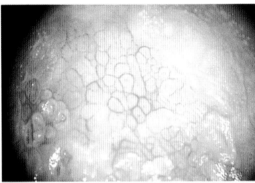

Plate 2 The atypical transformation zone: mosaic vascular pattern.

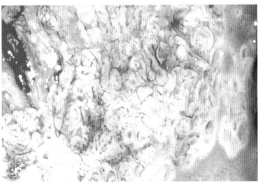

Plate 3 The atypical transformation zone: punctation.

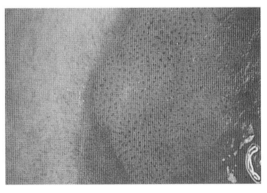

Plate 4 The atypical transformation zone: highly atypical vessels.

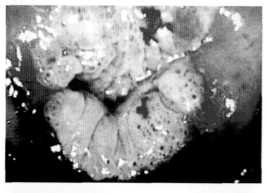

Plate 5 Early stromal invasion: coarse vascular pattern.

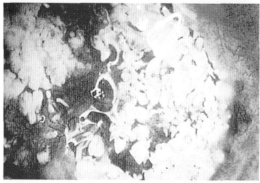

Plate 6 Microinvasion: dense aceto-white with coarse punctation and wide intercapillary distance.

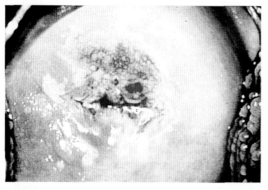

Plate 7 Microinvasion: irregular surface, dense acetowhite with coarse vessels.

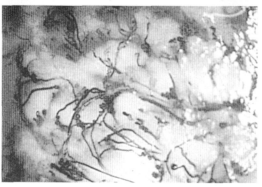

Plate 8 Invasion: abnormal vasculature—"corkscrew" and "comma".

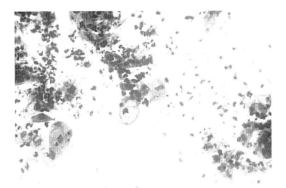

Plate 9 Inflammatory cervical cytology: background leukocytes may obscure and hinder correct interpretation. There are minimal nuclear changes.

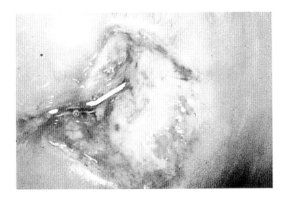

Plate 10 Primary syphilis of the cervix: the chancre would probably be misdiagnosed as squamous carcinoma at colposcopy. It is vegetative and friable, but possesses no typical characteristics.

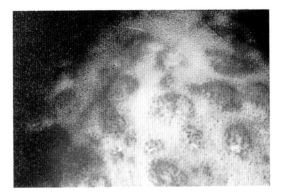

Plate 11 "Strawberry patches" of *Trichomonas vaginalis*: high power. This condition may be diagnosed by cytology or by typical symptomatology. The cervix often bleeds to the touch. Epithelial capillaries appear as clusters of red spots or "strawberry patches".

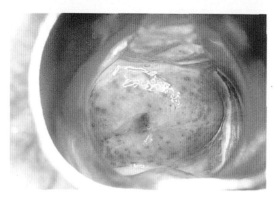

Plate 12 "Strawberry patches" of *Trichomonas vaginalis*: naked eye.

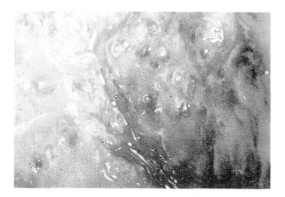

Plate 13 *Herpes simplex*: high power. Colposcopy shows vesicles, inflammation and ulceration of the cervix. Cytology may show typical "foam cells".

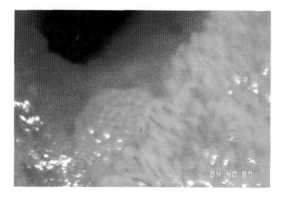

Plate 14 Human papillomavirus (HPV): high power. Colposcopy shows raspberry-like "asperities".

on cervical cytology include HPV, HSV, *Trichomonas vaginalis*, *Gardnerella vaginalis*, *Actinomyces* and possibly *Chlamydia trachomatis*. Cervical cytology, however, is not a screening tool for infection, nor a replacement for appropriate history taking and microscopic/microbiological testing.

Likewise, sexually transmitted diseases are not in themselves an indication for colposcopy, but may be present. The following text briefly describes their colposcopic characteristics, but the reader should refer to a good atlas of colposcopy for pictorial reference.

Syphilis

The cervix is the sole site of primary ulceration in only 5% of cases. The ulcer is usually mistaken for squamous cell carcinoma, but genital herpes, chancroid, tuberculosis, lymphogranuloma venereum and Behçet's disease should also be considered, as well as an infected injury or drug-induced eruption (Plate 10). The lesion may be vegetative, but possesses no typical characteristics.

Trichomonas vaginalis

The cervix may be seen to bleed to the touch. Colposcopic examination shows a background inflammatory picture with small epithelial capillaries appearing as clusters of red spots (Plates 11, 12). These are caused by loss of the superficial layers of the squamous epithelium and can appear on the cervix and/or vagina, being described as the 'strawberry cervix'. A 'leopard-skin' appearance can occur after challenge with iodine.

Candida albicans

Candida produces an intense inflammatory response, with the epithelium of the cervix and vagina thickening and becoming covered with a curdy, creamy-white discharge. Plaques adherent to the epithelium may bleed when disturbed, but should wipe away with saline on a swab stick, rarely interfering with colposcopic examination.

Herpes genitalis infection

The cervix is rarely the sole site of ulceration. The diagnosis will usually be suggested by a typical history and clinical presentation. Colposcopic changes may be evident in the form of vesicles and epithelial inflammation, which is caused by cellular infiltration just prior to ulceration (Plate 13).

The small vesicles seen early in the infection do not last long, ulcerating and coalescing to produce the more usual appearance of a single, serpiginous herpetic ulcer.

A constellation of symptomatology, history, viral culture and appearance can avoid the use of cervical biopsy to exclude malignancy. 'Foam cells' on cytology are very specific.

Spontaneous resolution without scarring is usual and this is hastened by appropriate antiviral therapy.

Human papillomavirus

The appearance colposcopically of exophytic condylomata is varied but their appearance on the cervix or vagina only, without external genital lesions, is unusual.

Before the application of acetic acid, condylomata are soft, poorly defined tumours, often resembling small raspberries in colour and form, but may be pink or white. They are composed of fine, finger-like projections, each with a central capillary, which tends to be obscured when the papillae whiten after the application of acetic acid (the so-called 'asperities') (Plate 14).

The presence of exophytic cervical warts is an indication for colposcopy in order to determine the presence or absence of lesions in other sites, any associated CIN/VaIN and to differentiate from the rare condylomatous carcinoma, which is an invasive squamous cell carcinoma integrated with condylomata acuminata.

The appearance of subclinical HPV on the cervix is mentioned elsewhere in this book.

Other pathogens

Endocervical mucopus and hypertrophic cervicitis are said to be associated with *Chlamydia trachomatis* infection. Immature metaplasia can be found also, as it can with Cytomegalovirus.

WOMEN WITH HUMAN IMMUNODEFICIENCY VIRUS (HIV)

Invasive cervical cancer in the presence of HIV infection has recently been added to the list of illnesses that define AIDS (acquired immune deficiency syndrome). Whether the sole mechanism for the association is immune depletion or not is as yet unclear. The higher prevalence of CIN in immunosuppressed women, such as those with renal transplants, supports the view that impaired immune surveillance facilitates oncogenesis. Women infected with HIV may be at higher risk of developing cervical cancer independently of HIV infection, because of other risk factors.

Despite the risk for HIV-positive women, however, deaths due to cervical cancer are rare, probably because premature morbidity due to other manifestations of AIDS occurs before the onset of extensive cervical disease.

Management of such women, therefore, must be a compromise and attempt to balance the increased risk of developing cervical neoplasia with the need to avoid as far as possible, adding to the psychological and physical trauma that such women face.

Women who are HIV-positive should be offered initial cytological and colposcopic screening to identify CIN. In those women who are found to have abnormal smears or CIN, CD4 lymphocyte counts should be monitored as usual.

Annual cytology with early recourse to diagnostic colposcopy is recommended, particularly in the presence of clinical immunosuppression, HIV-related disease and/or a CD4 count of less than 200. While regular colposcopic examination has been advocated, its benefits are not clear.

Any treatment required must not be denied the patient on the sole grounds of HIV positivity.

MANAGEMENT OF CIN IN GUM CLINICS

The advantages of 'in house' treatment and/or colposcopy are as follows.

1. Counselling

A woman who is already a patient will have her cytology explained to her, probably at a subsequent routine clinic visit. Face-to-face discussion and explanation of the need for colposcopy can be detailed. This may extend to an introduction to the colposcopy situation and equipment to help allay fears.

2. Continuity of care

Colposcopy and treatment can be performed in the same setting and by the same staff already known to the patient.

3. Confidentiality

The advantages of restricting an individual's sensitive medical information to the least number of people and case-notes is obvious. It is not contradictory to note, however, that disclosure of personal details to the FHSA computer database and general practitioner can also be to the patient's advantage.

The case for and against disclosure can be put to the woman and appropriate counselling should result in the correct solution for that individual.

4. Shorter waiting times

When patients are referred internally only, colposcopy and treatment clinics are smaller and waiting times tend to be shorter. This is a definite encouragement to attend. Some clinics perform colposcopy, as results become known, during routine clinics.

5. Fail-safe and defaulter follow-up

Some women fail to provide their correct personal details when they attend GUM clinics. Others express the wish for their results, including cervical cytology, to be kept from their general practitioner. Some women request that no form of written and/or telephone contact is made from the clinic.

It can be seen from the above that there is a potential for breakdown in communication, failure to disclose information and potential problems of follow-up for GUM colposcopy patients. This tends not to be the case, however, since the above limitations are true of every-day STD management and, with the intervention of a health adviser, potential problems can be avoided.

GUM clinics should have a fail-safe procedure that takes account of the above. This must include increased commitment where correct information or communication is lacking or denied.

In reality, default rates from colposcopy clinics in GUM are lower than in standard gynaecological colposcopy practice, probably because of the familiarity with, and acceptance of, the above problems.

CIN TREATMENT IN GUM CLINICS: CONCLUSIONS

Treatment of CIN 'in house' recognizes the concept of continuation of care. The GUM physician must be trained in colposcopy and treatment methodologies, and a theoretical and practical knowledge of the diagnosis and management of other pelvic pathologies is invaluable. Likewise, gynaecologists will benefit from a basic understanding of the management of STDs and close collaboration with their GUM colleagues.

Local methods of treatment are associated with primary and secondary haemorrhage in a small number of cases and a few patients will require hospital admission. Close collaboration with gynaecological colleagues, extending to common management protocols and interdisciplinary audit, are to be commended. Treatment should not be performed where the facilities for admission and resuscitation are not immediately available.

LEARNING POINTS

1. Sexually transmitted diseases are not an indication for colposcopy and cytology is not an infection screen. The presence of STDs may modify colposcopic appearances.

2. An increased frequency for cervical screening is not supported for the female GUM population on the grounds of sexual behaviour, age or history of sexually transmitted disease. Opportunistic screening is valuable and GUM clinics are ideally placed to implement it.
3. Diagnosis and treatment of CIN must be to high standards of quality, accuracy and safety wherever they may be performed. GUM colposcopists should be trained to recognize gynaecological diseases and gynaecologists should be aware of sexually transmitted diseases.
4. HIV positive women should have annual cytology performed where appropriate but management and treatment must not be denied on grounds of seropositivity alone.
5. Confidentiality may extend to non-disclosure of patients' names and other details to the laboratory, GP, etc. The advantages and disadvantages for the woman should be discussed with her and her wishes should be respected.

MCQS

44. The following statements regarding viral infections of the cervix are true:
    a. Wart virus infection reported on a cervical smear is an indication for colposcopy
    b. Cervical cytology is highly specific in diagnosing Herpes simplex virus
    c. Women with a past history of genital Herpes simplex virus should have annual cervical cytology
    d. Warts on the cervix stain white with acetic acid
    e. HPV 16 and 18 infection demonstrates an acetowhite response; HPV 6 and 11 do not

45. The following are true of sexually transmitted diseases:
    a. The 'strawberry cervix' is suggestive of *Trichomonas vaginalis* infection
    b. *Gardnerella vaginalis* causes irregular branching of subepithelial capillaries, giving a classical colposcopic appearance
    c. The pathognomonic cytological indication of Herpes simplex virus is the 'foam cell'
    d. Exophytic cervical warts are an indication for annual cervical cytology
    e. 5% of deaths from squamous carcinoma of the cervix in the UK are in HIV-positive women

| 17 | **Counselling patients** |

P. Walker

INTRODUCTION

Interacting with the colposcopy services because of the identification of an abnormality on a cervical smear can be an exceedingly anxiety-provoking situation. Women have explained that the shock of hearing that they have had an abnormal result is compounded by a triple threat. They perceive a threat to their mortality because the word cancer has been used, a threat to their fertility because they assume treatment will adversely affect their reproductive potential and, finally, a challenge to their sexuality because cervical cancer itself is often referred to as 'a sexually transmitted disease'. It should be the aim of everyone involved in the cervical screening programme to adopt strategies to allay these anxieties.

Generally speaking, psychologists recognize two types of coping strategy in people involved in medical treatment. For one group their anxiety is compounded by the lack of information; these patients are called 'monitors'. In the colposcopy situation, if these women are given information at all stages, often in considerable detail, many of their anxieties will be relieved. The other or opposite group are called 'blunters'. For these women too much information, especially of a detailed and medically orientated type, will actually worsen their anxiety. In different societies and in different parts of society the relative proportions of these two groups will vary, but the provision of information at all stages of the screening and treatment cycle, adapted for local usage, is essential.

Handbook of Colposcopy, edited by David Luesley, Mahmood Shafi and Joe Jordan. Published in 1996 by Chapman & Hall, London. ISBN 0 412 71550 3

INFORMATION AT THE SCREENING SMEAR

In many ways, the best time to explain the real significance of an abnormal result is at the time the test itself is performed. It should be explained to the woman that, whereas it is expected that nine times out of 10, her smear will be normal, as many as one in 10 women will be recalled either because the smear shows an abnormality, about a 1 in 50 chance, or because it is technically unsatisfactory for reporting, about a 1 in 12 chance. The chance of a smear identifying invasive cancer in an asymptomatic woman is about 1 in 1000. Therefore, it is best to say to the woman that if she should receive a letter saying the smear result is unsatisfactory, the most likely scenario is either that it simply needs to be repeated for technical reasons, there could be a minor change that needs checking in 6 months or so, or there is a slight possibility that the cervix needs a slightly closer look with a magnifying glass; there is almost no possibility that an abnormal result means cancer. This message, stated at screening and reinforced if necessary by an information sheet, should help all women who later receive an abnormal result letter. Of crucial importance is that everyone in the practice or clinic – doctor, nurse and receptionist – should understand these figures and the relative risks involved so that a consistent message is imparted.

INFORMATION ABOUT COLPOSCOPY

It has been demonstrated that the anxiety experienced by women sitting waiting for a colposcopy examination is higher than that measured in women in hospital the night before major gynaecological surgery. Much of the anxiety can be alleviated if the patient receives, with the details of her appointment, an information booklet explaining in simple terms what the procedure involves and why it is being performed. In the early days of colposcopy, such booklets prepared by well-intentioned support groups often inadvertently worsened anxiety. The original booklets would contain on the same page a description of cryotherapy and a description of radical surgery and radiotherapy. It has been found that a simple booklet written in lay person's terms, not in too much detail, is much more effective. The most successful information booklets are those that are personalized to the individual clinic, with a photograph of the hospital or unit and, if possible, of current members of the nursing staff so that the patient will recognize a friendly face when she attends. These fact sheets must also contain a few words reinforcing the point that the condition is minor, suitable for local treatment, often as an outpatient, and carries little, if any, risk to potential fertility.

In the psychology studies performed one important fact was recognized and was a little surprising to the clinicians. Whereas, of course, the anxiety of the woman waiting for colposcopy was to a certain degree related to the disease process, an equal quotient was an anxiety about the performance of the procedure itself. One booklet contains the following advice to women on this issue:

Before the examination

You may find it helpful to bring a friend with you. The examination is carried out in a room in the outpatients department. You will first meet a nurse who will take you in to see the gynaecologist. In the room after talking to the gynaecologist, you'll be asked to go behind the curtains and undress from the waist downwards. Before the examination the nurse will help you position yourself on the couch and ensure that your legs are comfortable in the leg rests. The procedure will last 10-15 minutes so shuffle around to make sure you are comfortable and can stay in that position for the length of the examination.

The examination

At the start of the examination the doctor will take a smear in the same way as your general practitioner. After this the doctor will look at your cervix using the colposcope. This is not painful. No anaesthetic is needed and you will be conscious throughout the whole examination. In order to see any abnormal area the doctor will apply some liquids. The first is vinegar (this may sting a little). As a final check the doctor may apply a brown liquid (iodine). The doctor may want to take a very small sample of tissue in order to look at an area more carefully. This is a biopsy and may feel slightly painful.

After the examination

First get dressed. The doctor will usually be able to tell you what the problem is, if any. If there is a problem, this will be explained to you and if you need treatment what and when this should be done.

What can I do to make the examination easier?

Remember

1 in 12 women have an abnormal smear so it is far from being a rare problem. Colposcopy is a simple, quick and painless procedure.

When on the couch

Make sure you are comfortable. Shuffle your bottom to the edge of the couch. Make sure your legs are comfortable on the leg rests before the examination starts.

How to feel less nervous

1. Remember the doctor and nurse want to make the examination as easy as possible for you, so feel free to talk to the doctor or nurse. Ask any questions you want to, however silly they may seem.
2. Take deep breaths. Focus on relaxing. As you breathe out try and imagine the tension draining out of your body.
3. People find different things helpful when dealing with difficult situations. Some people find it helpful to focus on what is happening during the examination. Ask the doctor or nurse to tell you everything as it happens, if this could be helpful for you. Focus on the sensations that you are feeling at each stage of the examination.

    Other people find it helpful to distract themselves from what is happening during the examination. To do this choose an enjoyable daydream (such as lying on a tropical beach!). Describe everything in the daydream in great detail including all the sights, sounds and smells around you.

If you have any questions or worries ask the clinic staff: they are there to help you.

Reproduced from *Your Visit to the Royal Free Hospital Colposcopy Clinic*, published by the Patient Information Department of the Royal Free Hampstead NHS Trust, London

INFORMATION AT COLPOSCOPY

However well prepared the patient is as a result of adequate information having been provided at screening and with her appointment, at the colposcopy visit, the doctor will wish to explain, to all except the most vehement of blunters, the basic physiology of metaplasia and the natural history of cervical intraepithelial neoplasia. Many will employ diagrams but apart from a basic template of the uterus, cervix and vagina, it has been found most effective to draw on the template in front of the patient at the time of the consultation, rather than to have a series of previously prepared sheets. Terminology is very important and some lay terms are in frequent use in this situation: neck of the womb for cervix, soft and hard cells for endocervical and squamous cells, changing area for transformation zone and so on. The opportunity must be taken to state again the positive aspects of having been identified at this extremely early stage, that the woman does not have cancer, her fertility will not be affected and her sexuality is in no way being challenged.

There is little doubt that most patients with CIN 3 and CIN 2 who are not pregnant will be advised to undergo treatment. As well as details about the treatment itself, which will be discussed below, it is important to stress that, untreated, between 30% and 70% of women with CIN 3 will progress to invasive cancer whereas once treated less than 4 in 1000 will do so in a lifetime. Important though treatment reasonably soon is, however, it should be mentioned that the mean length of time for CIN 3 to become invasive is about 7–8 years. This additional information rather than encouraging delay simply balances the medical imperative for treatment at a measured pace and will deflect worry that the patient thinks she may have or is about to get cancer itself.

As most will accept, the situation with regard to CIN 1 is far less clear-cut. The patient will need to make her own decision on the evidence that only 14% of CIN 1 lesions progress to CIN 3, let alone cancer, whereas 86% will remain at the level of CIN 1 or regress completely over 10 years. She will need to balance the possibilities of the conservative approach against the disadvantage of non-treatment, which entails 6-monthly colposcopic visits, possibly for some years ahead. It is probable that the patient will make this decision based on her own assessment of the relative merits of the case for her as an individual and it is the role of her doctor simply to provide her with accurate information and direct her decision-making only if requested so to do.

INFORMATION ABOUT TREATMENT

Information sheets about treatment were amongst the first patient fact sheets introduced in many colposcopy clinics. Certain key points should be covered (Fig. 17.1). It is important to stress that the treatment is minor, common up and down the country and successful. Most would tell their patients about a 95% first-time treatment success rate with resort to further treatment for the minority, this usually involving a second simple treatment rather than anything more drastic. It should be stated that most treatments are performed under local anaesthesia but that some women require and others may request a short, day-case general anaesthetic instead. Most importantly, information will be required about the possibility, type, nature and severity of bleeding postoperatively and this should be described in terms the woman can understand.

Most but perhaps not all, would advise their patients not to use tampons and to avoid penetrative vaginal intercourse for 4 weeks after treatment and if this is the local advice it should be in the leaflet. It is vital that the fact sheet contains contact names and contact numbers which the patients can use if they are worried about an expected or unexpected side effect or symptom during the recovery period. There should ideally be a telephone line devoted to this use only, with additional information about what to do and who to contact out of hours and at weekends. Finally, the precise nature of the follow-up protocol should be described and the importance of follow-up stressed. Interestingly, it is quite easy to place all this information on one sheet of A4 paper.

Dear

Laser treatment is a method of destroying abnormal tissue by evaporation. In your particular case, this means taking away the abnormal area on the neck of the womb with a 95% chance of cure with just one treatment. Occasionally, a shorter second treatment may be required. Treatment can be carried out in Out Patients with a local anaesthetic or occasionally, as an In Patient under general anaesthesia.

There is very little discomfort associated with the treatment, some experience a period-like pain, which goes away as soon as the treatment is completed.

Following laser treatment, one or two points must be observed:

1) Please DO NOT take any severe exercise for TEN DAYS.

2) For the first four weeks following treatment, DO NOT place anything in the vagina, i.e., no douching, no tampons and do not have intercourse.

3) You may experience some bleeding following therapy. This may not start for a few days and may last as long as two weeks. The bleeding may be anything from slight spotting to a flow as heavy as an average period. If the bleeding persists after two weeks or is so heavy as to cause you to change a max-pad every two hours or more, or if you are worried in any way, then please ring xxxxxxxx and a gynaecological sister will be able to advise you. Only three women in every hundred actually require any extra treatment because of heavy bleeding.

4) Laser therapy requires follow up. You will be given an appointment for a simple check up for six weeks following treatment and also an appointment for a repeat smear at six months after treatment. Following one further smear six months later, then we hope that you will then simply have to attend for an annual cervical smear.

5) Happily, a single laser treatment has no adverse effect on future fertility, pregnancy or labour.

* * * * * * * *

Fig. 17.1 A typical patient information sheet.

COMMON PATIENT CONCERNS

However thorough the information sheets, however talented as communicators the doctors and nurses may be, unfortunately many patients will be left with unanswered questions and they must be encouraged to articulate these.

Sex and promiscuity

There has been much, in fact, too much attention paid in the medical and the lay press to the possible sexually transmitted nature of cervical cancer and its precursors. As a result many women feel embarrassed and worried about the implications of this. Reassurance can be given to one group in particular by stating that 15% of cervical cancer is a glandular condition which, as far as we know, has nothing whatever to do with sexual behaviour. Although squamous cancer only occurs in women who are or have been sexually active, it must be stressed again and again that squamous cancer itself and CIN can and do affect those with unimpeachable reputations as well as those whom from time to time society may define as promiscuous. The diagnosis of CIN says nothing about a woman, her behaviour, her number of partners or their behaviour and this is precisely why such questions should never be asked of women at colposcopy, except and unless a clearly defined research study has been identified and approved. As far as the individual woman is concerned, her sexuality and behaviour are nothing to do with colposcopy or her colposcopist.

Viruses and partners

It is possible that human papillomavirus, in particular HPV type 16, may have an important role in the aetiology of cervix cancer. Unfortunately, this has led cytology laboratories to report the finding of koilocytosis as 'wart virus infection', on the smear report. This is unhelpful and unnecessary but continues and causes great concern to women. It is reasonable to say to women that the smear is not a test for a virus, which can only be identified in specialist laboratories using sophisticated DNA technology, and therefore she has not even had a test for a virus at all. In addition, it is true to say that the virus is very common – non-type-specific testing for the virus would find it in up to 70% or more of currently sexually active women. The virus usually does nothing; it may cause warts in some people which can be unaesthetic but which are amenable to treatment; and in only a few women does the virus appear to set the CIN train in motion. This, of course, once identified can easily be treated. The woman may be concerned that she will give the virus to her partner. Gently, her advisor must address the issue, if forced on the point, and say that her partner has already been exposed to it and may have been exposed to it before their relationship – after all most people are – and in any case, apart from visible warts if they are present, the man is in no danger. The presence of koilocytosis on a cervical smear is almost certainly not a reason for a woman to consider altering her sexual behaviour.

Contraception and pregnancy

There is no indication for a woman to be advised to change her method of contraception, except perhaps for the small group who have been investigated and treated for adenocarcinoma-*in-situ*, where some caution may be needed in those wishing to take oral oestrogen (as the role of steroid hormones remains largely unexplored in this situation). There is no need to recommend the use of barrier contraception in women with CIN or those who have been treated for it.

Future fertility

There is no evidence that a single treatment for CIN by a locally destructive or non-knife-cone biopsy local excisional technique has any adverse effect on a woman's future fertility, pregnancy, carriage or delivery. It is to be hoped that the same will prove to be the case for those treated twice with these methods but, as yet, there are no data available.

CIN in pregnancy (see also Chapter 15)

There is no reason to treat CIN in pregnancy provided the preinvasive nature of the lesion has been confirmed by an expert colposcopist. There is no evidence that the CIN process is accelerated by pregnancy, the only delay that occurs is delay in treatment until after delivery. CIN is not affected by vaginal delivery and CIN and even HPV (as far as we know) have absolutely no adverse effect on the fetus or baby.

These clear and simple messages should be reinforced for all women.

SUMMARY

Great care is required in counselling women about colposcopy and CIN. Information booklets personalized to the unit and expressed in simple terms, preferably with input in design from previous and current patients, can allay many of the anxieties women feel when they have an abnormal smear.

LEARNING POINTS

1. Many women experience anxiety as a result of cervical screening and interaction with colposcopy services because the diagnosis of an abnormal smear presents potential threats to their sexuality, fertility and mortality.

2. Much of the anxiety associated with the screening programme and colposcopy can be alleviated providing patients are provided with adequate information in written form supported by verbal explanation at all points in the process.

3. The true natural history of viral-associated minor epithelial abnormalities of the cervix remains unclear.

MCQS

46. Counselling women:
   a. Less anxiety is found in women waiting for a colposcopy examination than in those awaiting hysterectomy
   b. Women should be told that cancer of the cervix is a sexually transmitted disease
   c. Simple fact sheets rather than detailed booklets are more effective in reducing anxiety
   d. A monitoring coping strategy is aided by the provision of information
   e. The large majority of women with CIN 1 left untreated would not develop cervical cancer

Appendix A: FIGO staging of cervical cancer

Stage I: The carcinoma is strictly confined to the cervix (extension to the corpus should be disregarded)

Stage IA: Invasive cancer identified only microscopically. All gross lesions, even with superficial invasion, are stage 1B cancers.

Invasion is limited to measured stromal invasion with a maximum depth of 5 mm and no wider than 7 mm.*

Stage IA1: Measured invasion of stroma no greater than 3 mm in depth and no wider than 7 mm.

Stage IA2: Measured invasion of stroma greater than 3 mm and no greater than 5 mm in depth and no wider than 7 mm.

Stage IB: Clinical lesions confined to the cervix or preclinical lesions greater than IA

Stage IB1: Clinical lesions no greater than 4 cm in size.

Stage IB2: Clinical lesions greater than 4 cm in size.

Stage II: The carcinoma extends beyond the cervix, but has not extended on to the pelvic wall. The carcinoma involves the vagina, but not as far as the lower third.

Stage IIA: No obvious parametrial involvement.

Stage IIB: Obvious parametrial involvement.

Stage III: The carcinoma has extended on to the pelvic wall. On rectal examination there is no cancer-free space between the tumour and the pelvic wall.

The tumour involves the lower third of the vagina. All cases with a

*The depth of invasion should not be more than 5 mm taken from the base of the epithelium, either surface or glandular, from which it originates. Vascular space involvement, whether venous or lymphatic, should not alter the staging.

hydronephrosis or non-functioning kidney should be included, unless they are known to be due to other cause.

Stage IIIA: No extension on to the pelvic wall, but involvement of the lower third of the vagina.

Stage IIIB: Extension on to the pelvic wall or hydronephrosis or non-functioning kidney.

Stage IV: The carcinoma has extended beyond the true pelvis or has clinically involved the mucosa of the bladder or rectum.

Stage IVA: Spread of the growth to adjacent organs.

Stage IVB: Spread to distant organs.

Appendix B: Colposcopic terminology and technique

TERMINOLOGY

Histological terms

Original squamous epithelium is the squamous epithelium that is laid down at the time of organogenesis. Usually it covers the vagina and most of the ectocervix.

Original columnar epithelium refers to columnar epithelium laid down at the time of organogenesis. It is usually confined to the endocervical canal but commonly covers part of the ectocervix.

Metaplasia refers to the process by which columnar epithelium is replaced by squamous epithelium. It is stressed that this is a physiological process which occurs to a greater or lesser degree in all women. That part of the cervix which has been the site of metaplasia is recognizable colposcopically and is called the transformation zone.

Squamocolumnar junction is the line of demarcation between columnar and squamous epithelium.

Leukoplakia is a condition in which normal squamous epithelium is covered by a superficial cornified layer without visible nuclei. It is sometimes called **hyperkeratosis**.

Carcinoma-*in-situ* is a lesion that exhibits atypical cells throughout the whole thickness of the squamous epithelium. Individually these cells are indistinguishable from those of invasive carcinoma but they do not breach the basement membrane, i.e. there is no invasion.

Dysplasia represents a range of histological abnormalities between normal squamous epithelium and carcinoma-*in-situ*. The superficial cells are matured and fully differentiated but the underlying cells show atypical changes. Dysplasia is usually graded into mild, moderate and severe.

Cervical intraepithelial neoplasia (CIN) is a new classification which many investigators find easier to use than dysplasia and carcinoma-*in-situ*. One of its main advantages is that it removes the word carcinoma-*in-situ* from the terminology. There are three grades of CIN:

CIN I: equivalent to mild to moderate dysplasia;

CIN II: an intermediate grade;

CIN III: equivalent to severe dysplasia or carcinoma-*in-situ*.

Microinvasive carcinoma is used if there is a minor degree of invasion. There is no generally accepted definition for this lesion but most histopathologists would use the term if invasion was less than 4–5 mm below the basement membrane.

Invasive carcinoma is present when there is unquestionable invasion by malignant cells.

Colposcopic terms

Acetowhite epithelium: When 3% or 5% acetic acid is applied to the cervix, abnormal epithelium becomes white, with a sharp line of demarcation between the abnormal epithelium and the normal epithelium, which remains pink. In other words, acetowhite epithelium refers to that epithelium which is white **after** the application of acetic acid, in contradistinction to **leukoplakia**, which is white **before** the application of acetic acid.

Leukoplakia or **hyperkeratosis** refers to epithelium that is white before the application of acetic acid. This can be seen with the naked eye.

Erosion is mentioned here because, although it does not form part of the colposcopic terminology, it is commonly used in gynaecology. Colposcopic assessment of the cervix will show that a true erosion is an extremely rare occurrence, and when the gynaecologist describes the cervix as being the site of an erosion s/he usually means that it is red because of the presence of an ectopy (see below) or inflammation.

Ectopy is used to denote the presence of columnar epithelium on the ectocervix. Such a cervix will appear red, particularly in pregnant women or those using the combined oral contraceptive, and a firmly taken cervical smear will often produce bleeding. An ectopy is not an abnormal finding and does not require treatment unless it is causing symptoms such as postcoital bleeding or excessive vaginal discharge.

Squamocolumnar junction (SCJ) is the easily recognized junction between squamous epithelium (whether normal or abnormal) and columnar epithelium.

Typical transformation zone (TTZ): This is the most important part of the cervix as far as the colposcopist is concerned. It refers to that part of the cervix which has been transformed by a process of metaplasia from columnar epithelium to squamous epithelium. The transformation zone can be quite easily recognized by the presence of small gland openings, small

Nabothian follicles and a typical subepithelial capillary pattern. It is important that the colposcopist should always inspect the transformation zone early and become familiar with its recognition. If the transformation zone is normal it is called 'typical transformation zone', whereas if there is any suggestion of abnormality it is called 'atypical transformation zone'.

Atypical transformation zone (ATZ) refers to a transformation zone that shows epithelium with the characteristics of abnormality. The colposcopist would suspect the presence of abnormal epithelium if s/he sees the following:

1. leukoplakia (hyperkeratosis);
2. acetowhite epithelium;
3. an abnormal subepithelial capillary pattern – punctation, mosaic or atypical vessels.

TECHNIQUE OF COLPOSCOPY

Several types of colposcopy are available but all have the same basic property: to view the cervix at magnifications varying from × 6 to × 40. For colposcopy to be performed, the patient is placed in a modified lithotomy position. The cervix is exposed with a bivalve speculum following which the epithelium is inspected. There are two basic schools of colposcopy, that using classical or extended colposcopy and that using the saline technique; most people belong to the former.

Classical or extended colposcopy

This is the method advocated by the German school and is practised at most colposcopy centres. The cervix and upper vagina are first examined at magnifications of × 6, × 10 and × 16, following which excess mucus is removed from the cervix with a dry cotton wool swab and the cervix is again inspected. If it is thought necessary to take a cervical smear it should be done at this stage, care being taken not to be too vigorous in the scraping, otherwise bleeding may occur and cause difficulties in interpreting the colposcopic findings. Routine smear-taking at the first visit is not always necessary because the colposcopist usually already knows that the cytology is abnormal – hence the referral to the colposcopy clinic.

Acetic acid test

Acetic acid (3% or 5%) is gently applied by means of a cotton wool swab. The acetic acid is held in place for about 5 seconds, following which it is relatively easy to remove most of any remaining mucus. Abnormal epithelium, if present, now appears white (acetowhite epithelium) and almost invariably is very easy to distinguish from normal epithelium because of a sharp line of demarcation between the two. The normal squamous epithelium appears pink because the light from the colposcope picks up the redness of the subepithelial capillary pattern. Abnormal epithelium is white because the acetic acid coagulates protein in the nuclei and the cytoplasm; abnormal epithelium has a high nuclear density and therefore a high concentration of protein. This prevents light from passing through, the end result being that the subepithelial vessel pattern is less easy to see and the epithelium appears white. The higher the concentration of protein the more intense will be the white appearance. The effect of the acetic acid wears off after about 30–40 seconds but reappears after a further application. Following the application of the acetic acid, Schiller's iodine may be applied.

Schiller's iodine test

Normal squamous epithelium is characterized by an abundance of glycogen whereas abnormal epithelium has relatively little. Application of Lugol's iodine solution to normal squamous epithelium will therefore produce a dark brown, almost black stain while columnar epithelium and abnormal epithelium, which contain little or no glycogen, remain unstained. Most experienced colposcopists do not use the Schiller's iodine test although for the trainee colposcopist it is essential as occasionally milder forms of abnormality will be seen that would otherwise have remained undetected.

Saline technique

Because the use of acetic acid or Lugol's iodine makes it difficult to study the angioarchitecture of the cervix, the saline technique was devised by Koller and developed by Kolstad, both working from the Norwegian Radium Hospital in Oslo. After the cervix has been exposed, mucus is gently removed with a cotton wool swab and the cervix is moistened with physiological saline, which allows the subepithelial angioarchitecture to be studied in great detail. To see the capillaries clearly the use of a green filter and high magnification is advised, thus making the red capillaries appear darker and therefore stand out more clearly. The technique depends entirely on visualization of various vessel patterns and, although it is a much more difficult technique to master, it allows the colposcopist to predict the underlying histological pattern with great accuracy.

NORMAL AND ABNORMAL COLPOSCOPIC APPEARANCES

There are certain predictable features which the colposcopist must assess following the application of acetic acid and these can be summarized as follows:

1. vascular pattern;
2. intercapillary distance;
3. colour tone relative to the junction of normal and abnormal tissue;
4. surface pattern;
5. sharp line of demarcation between different types of epithelium.

Of these criteria probably the most important are the vascular pattern and the intercapillary distance, and it is important that the colposcopist is thoroughly familiar with the different types of capillary that can be observed in the surface epithelium of normal and abnormal cervical epithelium.

Vascular pattern

Seen under the colposcope the vascular pattern of normal squamous epithelium appears as fine dots or as a network of fine capillaries. Abnormal epithelium, on the other hand, has capillaries which are described as either punctation vessels, mosaic vessels or atypical vessels.

Punctation is an easily recognized vascular pattern characterized by dilated, elongated and often twisted vessels arranged in a prominent punctate pattern.

Mosaic vessels are arranged parallel to the surface in a characteristic mosaic or 'crazy paving' pattern.

Atypical vessels are capillaries that are very easily seen by the colposcopist. Typically they are irregular in size, shape, course and arrangement.

Intercapillary distance

The intercapillary distance is the distance between vessels or the space encompassed by the mosaic vessels. The maximum intercapillary distance of normal capillaries varies but is approximately 50–250 μm with an average of 100 μm. Colposcopic assessment of the intercapillary distance in abnormal epithelium is most easily done by comparing the abnormal capillaries with the capillaries of the adjacent normal squamous epithelium. The intercapillary distance in CIN and early invasive carcinoma of the cervix increases with the advancing grade of the lesion, i.e. in CIN I lesions the average intercapillary distance may be 200 μm whereas in CIN III it is often 450–550 μm.

Colour tone

When using the saline technique abnormal epithelium appears much darker than normal epithelium, whereas following the application of acetic acid abnormal epithelium appears very white (acetowhite epithelium). In both cases, particularly following the application of acetic acid, an easily recognizable sharp line of demarcation between normal and abnormal epithelium can be observed.

Surface pattern

The surface of the lesion can be described as being smooth and even, granular, papillomatous or nodular. Normal squamous epithelium, for example, has a smooth surface while columnar epithelium is easily recognized by its typical grape-like or villus appearance. At the other extreme invasive cancer is characterized by an uneven, nodular and often exophytic growth pattern.

Lines of demarcation

The line of demarcation between normal squamous epitehlium and abnormal epithelium is usually sharp as a result of the change in colour that is present in abnormal epithelium.

Appendix C: Basic colposcopy: multiple choice questions

All statements are either true or false.

CHAPTER 1

1. The ectocervical native epithelium is:
   a. Of columnar mucinous type   F
   b. Sensitive to hormone effects   T
   c. Of multilayered squamous type   T
   d. Commonly ulcerated   F
   e. Very fragile in comparison to the endocervical epithelium   F

2. The 'physiological' SCJ:
   a. Is where the squamous and endocervical epithelium met in
      childhood   F
   b. Is a fixed point   F
   c. Moves under the influence of hormones   T
   d. Is usually within the endocervical canal in the post-menopausal
      woman   T
   e. Doesn't exist   F

3. The transformation zone:
   a. Is where native endocervical epithelium has been converted to
      squamous epithelium   T
   b. Persists even into the post-menopausal years   T

    c. Never has underlying crypts   F
    d. Can be identified colposcopically by the presence of gland
       openings   T

4. Squamous metaplasia is
    a. A pathological process   F
    b. Brought about by the effect of vaginal acidity   T
    c. Stimulated by trauma   T
    d. Caused by Human papillomavirus   F
    e. Preceded by reserve cell hyperplasia   T

5. The congenital transformation zone is:
    a. Formed prenatally   T
    b. Related to uterine fundal abnormalities   F
    c. Disappears after the menopause   F
    d. Often associated with excess epithelial glycogen production   F
    e. Invisible colposcopically   F

CHAPTER 2

6. The following statements with regard to cervical smear-taking and
    reporting are true:
    a. The person taking the smear usually decides if the sample is
       adequate   F
    b. A smear report of moderate dyskaryosis should be managed as
       for mild dyskaryosis   F
    c. The transformation zone is difficult to sample in postmenopausal
       patients   T
    d. Colposcopy is not indicated following a smear report of abnormal
       endocervical cells   F
    e. Cervical cytology can reliably detect invasive squamous cell cancer   F

CHAPTER 3

7. The following histological features distinguish CIN 3 from CIN 1:
    a. CIN 3 shows greater nuclear pleomorphism than CIN 1   T
    b. CIN 3 shows greater variation in nuclear size than CIN 1   T
    c. CIN 3 shows better differentiation than CIN 1   F
    d. Nuclei at the surface are normal in CIN 1   F
    e. Nucleoli are more prominent in CIN 1 than in CIN 3   F

8. The following are histological features of early invasive carcinoma:
    a. Focal lymphocytic infiltrate in the stroma   T

b. Anaplasia of the invasive cells   F
c. Eosinophilia of the invasive cells   T
d. Ulceration of the surface epithelium   F
e. Focal condensation of stromal collagen   F

9. Which of the following statements about CIN are true?
    a. CIN naturally falls into three categories rather than two   F
    b. The term low-grade squamous intraepithelial lesion includes
       both CIN 1 and Human papillomavirus infection   T
    c. High-grade squamous intraepithelial lesion is an alternative
       name for CIN 2   T
    d. Cervical crypts may be involved by all grades of CIN   T
    e. Most examples of keratinizing CIN arise from the original
       squamous epithelium of the ectocervix   F

CHAPTER 4

10. With regard to the history of colposcopy:
    a. Colposcopy was introduced by Hans Hinselmann   T
    b. Colposcopy largely replaced cervical cytology   F
    c. Commonly used magnifications are up to 100-fold   F
    d. An understanding of histopathology is useful for practising
       colposcopists   T
    e. The green filter has been an important development in the field
       of colposcopy   T

11. With regard to equipment in the colposcopy clinic:
    a. A bivalve speculum is ideal to visualize the cervix   T
    b. Cervical smears should never be taken prior to colposcopy F
    c. Nitric acid is an important stain to detect preinvasive changes F
    d. An endocervical speculum is useful for examining the lower
       endocervical canal   T
    e. Biopsies should only be taken in exceptional circumstances F

12. During a colposcopic examination:
    a. The cervix should be fully exposed   T
    b. For a satisfactory colposcopic assessment, the squamocolumnar
       junction should be visualized   T
    c. Normal squamous epithelium fails to stain with Lugol's iodine F
    d. Areas of metaplasia are where the squamous epithelium is
       transforming to columnar epithelium   F
    e. Only abnormal epithelium turns white with the application of
       acetic acid   F

CHAPTER 5

13. In colposcopy of the normal cervix:
    a. It is possible to demonstrate three levels of metaplasia T
    b. The green filter was introduced by Lugol F
    c. The transformation zone can contain columnar epithelium T
    d. Metaplasia is smooth, confluent and regular F
    e. Double capillaries are suggestive of an inflammatory process T

14. At colposcopy, normal columnar epithelium:
    a. Demonstrates a red appearance because of subepithelial haemorrhage F
    b. Is characterized by a 'grape-like' appearance T
    c. Does not change following the application of 5% acetic acid F
    d. Has identifiable villi each with one central capillary T
    e. Shows microvilli on the surface of columnar cells F

CHAPTER 6

15. The following are indications for colposcopy in the UK:
    a. A single mildly dyskaryotic smear F
    b. A single moderately dyskaryotic smear T
    c. A single severely dyskaryotic smear T
    d. A cervical polyp F
    e. A routine follow-up visit 18 months after treatment for CIN 3 F

16. Which of the following statements about cervical smears are true?
    a. There is a high correlation between negative cytology and negative histology T
    b. There is a poor correlation between low-grade cytology and low-grade histology F
    c. There is a high correlation between high-grade cytology and high-grade histology T
    d. HPV 16 is a high-risk oncogenic virus T
    e. HPV 6 is a high-risk oncogenic virus F

17. Colposcopy:
    a. Was first developed in Germany T
    b. Is used as a screening tool in some genito-urinary medicine clinics in the UK T
    c. Is usually performed at a magnification of × 40 F
    d. Is only used to examine female anatomy F
    e. Is essential in the diagnosis of VIN F

CHAPTER 7

18. The transformation zone (TZ):
    a. Is delineated as the area below the SCJ   F
    b. That shows acetowhitening is pathognomonic of CIN   F
    c. That shows a mosaic pattern has low-grade CIN   F
    d. That shows diffuse punctation extending on to the original
       squamous epithelium suggests an inflammatory process   T
    e. Fine terminal vessel branching is not usually associated with
       atypical vessels   T

19. HPV infection:
    a. Is always clearly defined colposcopically   F
    b. Is not confined to the transformation zone   T
    c. Can have an encephaloid appearance   T
    d. Has clearly defined margins when seen colposcopically   F
    e. Can usefully be categorized by using scoring systems   F

20. Inflammatory changes:
    a. Are always associated with bacterial infection   F
    b. Can be caused by *Candida albicans*   T
    c. Are present in schistosomal infection   T
    d. May be similar to atrophic changes on colposcopy   F
    e. On colposcopy, the appearances are compatible with hyperaemia
       of the vascular bed   T

CHAPTER 8

21. With regard to subclinical invasive lesions of the cervix:
    a. The majority will be accurately diagnosed by colposcopy   F
    b. If suspected, formal knife cone biopsy is mandatory   F
    c. Leukoplakia is highly predictive that such lesions are present   F
    d. Abnormal vessels are highly suggestive   T
    e. Pregnancy changes may mask the usual colposcopic features   F

22. The following statements are true:
    a. When glandular lesions are suspected excisional biopsy must be
       performed   T
    b. When frank invasion is apparent diagnostic cone biopsy is
       mandatory   F
    c. Coarse punctation is a cardinal colposcopic feature of
       adenocarcinoma-*in-situ*   F
    d. Early invasive lesions are likely to have wide intercapillary
       distances   T
    e. Acetic acid application can mask abnormal vascular patterns   F

CHAPTER 9

23. Recording information in colposcopy clinics:
    a. When taking a history from a patient with an abnormal cervical smear it is important to ask about the age at first intercourse   F
    b. All patients having colposcopy should have a bimanual examination   F
    c. Invagination of the vaginal angles following hysterectomy makes image recording difficult   T
    d. It is unnecessary to record a gynaecological history at the time of colposcopy   F
    e. The use of digital image capture has no proven benefits in managing patients in the colposcopy clinic   T

24. In colpophotography:
    a. Hand-held 35 mm cameras give poorer quality photographs than those taken through the colposcope   T
    b. Black and white film (enhanced by the addition of a green filter) is better for recording vascular architecture   T
    c. Videophotography gives better depth of focus than still photography   F
    d. Cervicographs are assessed by an expert, who examines the final colour print of the cervix   F
    e. An objective lens of 400 mm is ideal for photographing the cervix   F

CHAPTER 10

25. Epidemiology:
    a. The all age incidence of cervical cancer is increasing   F
    b. Cervical cancer is the commonest female cancer   F
    c. Approximately 7% of all cervical smears taken are abnormal to some degree   T
    d. The commonest cytological abnormality is severe dyskaryosis   F
    e. Almost 5.5 million smears are performed annually in the UK   T

26. Patient selection:
    a. All cases of CIN must undergo immediate treatment   F
    b. Colposcopic opinion alone may not be enough if conservative management is being considered   T
    c. A directed punch biopsy will always give an accurate assessment of the degree of abnormality   F
    d. CIN in pregnancy should be immediately treated   F
    e. Age is a consideration in the management of low-grade lesions   T

27. Non-treatment of cytological abnormalities:
    a. If there is no lesion present at colposcopy and the cervical smear is normal a woman can safely be returned to the call and recall scheme   F
    b. Women with CIN 1 have a lower progressive potential than those with CIN 3   T
    c. HPV-associated lesions can be easily distinguished from CIN 1 on colposcopy   F
    d. HPV-associated changes are easily distinguished from CIN 1 on histological examination   F
    e. CIN has a centripetal distribution (i.e. higher-grade CIN is centrally placed in a lesion)   T

28. Colposcopy in pregnancy:
    a. Colposcopy and cervical smears may cause a miscarriage in early pregnancy   F
    b. Colposcopy is made easier in pregnancy due to hormonal effects on the cervix   F
    c. A punch biopsy is taken if CIN is suspected colposcopically   F
    d. Treatment of CIN may be deferred until the postnatal period   T
    e. If invasion is suspected, a wedge biopsy is taken for diagnostic purposes under general anaesthesia   T

29. Deferred management:
    a. Default rates may have an influence on deferred treatment strategies   T
    b. A transient population should be offered immediate treatment once CIN is diagnosed   T
    c. Peak incidence of low-grade lesions is between 35 and 40 years   F
    d. Stress levels return to normal immediately if the woman is offered deferred management   F
    e. The stress of colposcopy is similar to that of major surgery   T

CHAPTER 11

30. In the treatment of CIN:
    a. CIN 3 requires more radical treatment than CIN 1   F
    b. Colposcopy is required before any treatment method   T
    c. Before ablation, a directed biopsy should be performed   T
    d. Laser vaporization can be used to 'see and treat' without recourse to biopsy   F
    e. Local anaesthetic is not required for outpatient loop excision   F

31. The following are recognized complications of diathermy loop excision:
    a. Haemorrhage   T

    b. Pelvic inflammatory disease   F
    c. Cervical stenosis   T
    d. Infertility   F
    e. Dyspareunia   F

32. Treatment of CIN should not be performed:
    a. In pregnancy   T
    b. If there is an acute vaginal infection   T
    c. In the luteal phase   F
    d. During menstruation   F
    e. In women who are HIV-positive   F

CHAPTER 12

33. After local ablative or excisional treatment of CIN:
    a. The risk of frank invasive cancer is 1 in 1000   T
    b. Most residual disease will be recognized within 12 months   T
    c. Colposcopy and cytology should be performed within 3 months   F
    d. Recurrent disease is more likely than residual disease   F
    e. A success rate of between 90% and 95% can be expected   T

34. Follow-up for treated CIN:
    a. Includes colposcopy at 12 months in all women   F
    b. Is more likely to be abnormal in women who have had high-grade lesions treated   T
    c. Is based on colposcopy rather than cytology   F
    d. May be normal despite the presence of residual disease   T
    e. Requires an annual smear for three years   F

35. After a hysterectomy:
    a. Women who have never had an abnormal smear require no further cytological surveillance   T
    b. Colposcopy and cytology should be performed at 6 weeks   F
    c. Colposcopy and cytology should be a part of follow-up if CIN is present   T
    d. There is a risk of VaIN in all patients   F
    e. Lugol's iodine is more reliable in detecting residual CIN than acetic acid   F

36. In untreated patients with abnormal smears:
    a. Colposcopy may be normal despite a moderately dyskaryotic smear   T
    b. The preferred treatment for persistent dyskaryosis is ablation   F

c. Two consecutively negative smears are required prior to
   discharge back to routine recall T
d. Random punch biopsies should be performed if colposcopy is
   normal F
e. A normal punch biopsy means that the patient can be discharged
   to recall F

CHAPTER 13

37. Microinvasive cervical carcinoma:
    a. May be defined as a lesion visible on the cervix to the naked eye
       with a depth on invasion of 2 mm F
    b. May be cured by LLETZ T
    c. Carries a risk of nodal metastases of around 1% T
    d. May be defined as a lesion invading 3 mm or less below the
       basement membrane F

38. Adenocarcinoma of the cervix:
    a. Is increasing in incidence T
    b. Microinvasion is defined in terms of depth of invasion into the
       stroma from the nearest gland F
    c. Over 60% of cases of AIS coincide with *in-situ* or microinvasive
       squamous lesions T
    d. AIS treated by hysterectomy should include bilateral
       oophorectomy F

39. Pelvic lymphadenectomy should be considered:
    a. In cases of adenosquamous carcinoma-*in-situ* F
    b. In microinvasive cervical cancer with LVS invasion T
    c. For a lesion with a volume greater than 500 mm^3 T
    d. For a lesion invading 3 mm below the basement membrane F

40. Fertility may be conserved:
    a. With a microinvasive lesion 1–3 mm below the basement
       membrane T
    b. With a Stage Ia2 lesion T
    c. In a case of AIS T
    d. In a case of a mixed AIS/CIN lesion T

41. Cone biopsy alone can be considered curative in cases where:
    a. The depth of invasion is greater than 5 mm F
    b. The surface area of the lesion is greater than 50 mm^2 F
    c. The volume of the lesion is greater than 500 mm^3 F
    d. There is adenocarcinoma-*in-situ* T

CHAPTER 14

42. The following criteria are met by HPV screening:
    a. It is highly sensitive for all grades of cervical disease when performed in a qualitative manner   F
    b. The polymerase chain reaction is the most useful test in mass screening   F
    c. Medium/high copy numbers of HPV 16 can predict high-grade cervical disease more accurately than cervical cytology   T
    d. When assessed in a semiquantitative manner, screening may replace conventional cytology   F
    e. HPV types 16, 18, 31 and 33 are the most useful types to screen for in the UK   T

CHAPTER 15

43. During pregnancy
    a. CIN is more likely to progress to cancer   F
    b. The transformation zone becomes smaller   F
    c. CIN should be treated by laser   F
    d. Wedge biopsy is the preferred method of excluding invasion   T
    e. The endocervical speculum should not be used   F

CHAPTER 16

44. The following statements regarding viral infections of the cervix are true:
    a. Wart virus infection reported on the cervical smear is an indication for colposcopy   F
    b. Cervical cytology is highly specific in diagnosing Herpes simplex virus   F
    c. Women with a past history of genital Herpes simplex virus should have annual cervical cytology   F
    d. Warts on the cervix stain white with acetic acid   T
    e. HPV 16 and 18 infection demonstrates an acetowhite response; HPV 6 and 11 do not   F

45. The following are true of sexually transmitted diseases:
    a. The 'strawberry cervix' is suggestive of *Trichomonas vaginalis* infection   T
    b. *Gardnerella vaginalis* causes irregular branching of subepithelial capillaries, giving a classical colposcopic appearance   F
    c. The pathognomonic cytological indication of Herpes simplex virus is the 'foam cell'   T

d. Exophytic cervical warts are an indication for annual cervical
cytology   F
e. 5% of deaths from squamous carcinoma of the cervix in the UK
are in HIV-positive women   F

CHAPTER 17

46. Counselling women:
    a. Less anxiety is found in women waiting for a colposcopy
       examination than in those awaiting hysterectomy   F
    b. Women should be told that cancer of the cervix is a sexually
       transmitted disease   F
    c. Simple fact sheets rather than detailed booklets are more
       effective in reducing anxiety   T
    d. A monitoring coping strategy is aided by the provision of
       information   T
    e. The large majority of women with CIN 1 left untreated would
       not develop cervical cancer   T

Further reading

CHAPTER 1

Ferenczy, A. and Winkler, B. (1987) Anatomy and histology of the cervix, in *Pathology of the Female Genital Tract*, 3rd edn, (ed. R. Kurman), Springer, New York, p. 141.

Fu, Y. S. and Reagan, J. W. (1989) Development, anatomy and histology of the lower female genital tract, in *Pathology of the Uterine Cervix, Vagina and Vulva*, W. B. Saunders, Philadelphia, PA, p. 21.

Singer, A. and Jordan, J. A. (1976) The anatomy of the cervix, in *The Cervix*, (eds J. A. Jordan and A. Singer), W. B. Saunders, London, p. 141.

CHAPTER 2

Koss, L.G. (1989) The Papanicolaou test for cervical cancer: a triumph and a tragedy. *J. A. M. A.*, **261**, 734–743.

Evans, D. M. D., Hudson, E. A., Brown, C. L. *et al.* (1986) Terminology on gynaecological cytopathology: report of the working party of the BSCC. *J. Clin. Pathol.*, **39**, 933–944.

Wied, G. L., Keebler, C. M., Koss, L. G. *et al. (1992) Compendium of Diagnostic Pathology*, Tutorials of Cytology, Chicago, IL.

CHAPTER 3

Anderson, M. C. (1995) Premalignant and malignant squamous lesions of the cervix, in *Haines and Taylor Obstetrical and Gynaecological Pathology*, 4th edn, (eds H. Fox and M. Wells), Churchill Livingstone, Edinburgh, in press.

Anderson, M. C., Brown, C. L., Fox, H. *et al.* (1991) Current views on cervical intraepithelial neoplasia. *J. Clin. Pathol.*, **44**, 969–978.

Wright, T. C., Kurman, R. J. and Ferenczy, A. (1994) Precancerous lesions of the cervix, in *Blaustein's Pathology of the Female Genital Tract*, 4th edn, (ed. R. J. Kurman), Springer, New York.

CHAPTER 4

Jordan, J. A. (1985) Colposcopy in the diagnosis of cervical cancer and precancer. *Clin. Obstet. Gynecol.*, **12**, 67–76.
Soutter, W. P. (1991) Criteria for standards of management of women with an abnormal smear. *Br. J. Obstet. Gynaecol.*, **98**, 1069–1072.
Stafl, A. (1983) Understanding colposcopic patterns and their clinical significance. *Contemp. Obstet. Gynaecol.*, **21**, 85–104.

CHAPTER 6

Duncan, I. D. (1992) *Guidelines for Clinical Practice and Programme Management*, NHS Cervical Screening Programme National Co-ordinating Network, Oxford.
Jarmulowicz, M. R., Jenkins, D., Barton, S. E. *et al.* (1989) Cytological status and lesion size. A further dimension in cervical intraepithelial neoplasia. *Br. J. Obstet. Gynaecol.*, **96**, 1061–1106.
Jordan, J. A., Sharp, F. and Singer, A. (1981) *Preclinical Neoplasia of the Cervix: Proceedings of the 9th Study Group*, Royal College of Obstetricians and Gynaecologists, London.
Lyall, H. and Duncan, I. D. (1995) Inaccuracy of cytologic diagnosis in high grade squamous intraepithelial lesions (CIN 3). *Acta Cytol.*, **39**, 50–54.

CHAPTER 8

Anderson, M. C. (1993) Invasive carcinoma of the cervix following local destructive treatment for cervical intraepithelial neoplasia. *Br. J. Obstet. Gynaecol.*, **100**, 657–663.
Benedet, J., Anderson, G. and Boyes, D. (1985) Colposcopic accuracy in the diagnosis of microinvasive and occult invasive carcinoma of the cervix. *Obstet. Gynecol.*, **65**, 557–562.
Luesley, D., Cullimore, J., Redman, C. *et al.* (1990) Loop diathermy excision of the cervical transformation zone in patients with abnormal cervical smears. *Br. Med. J.*, **300**, 1690–1693.
Shafi, M., Finn, C., Luesley, D. *et al.* (1991) Lesion size and histology of atypical transformation zone. *Br. J. Obstet. Gynaecol.*, **98**, 490–492.
Shafi, M., Dunn, J., Chenoy, R. *et al.* (1994) Digital imaging colposcopy, image analysis, and quantification of the colposcopic image. *Br. J. Obstet. Gynaecol.*, **97**, 811–816.

CHAPTER 9

Shafi, M., Dunn, J., Chenoy, R. *et al.* (1994) Digital imaging colposcopy, image analysis, and quantification of the colposcopic image. *Br. J. Obstet. Gynaecol.*, **97**, 811–816.

Soutter, W. P. (1991) Criteria for standards of measurement of women with an abnormal smear. *Br. J. Obstet. Gynaecol.,* **98**, 1069–1072.

Stafl, A. (1981) Cervicography: a new method for cervical cancer detection. *Am. J. Obstet. Gynecol.,* **139**, 815–825.

CHAPTER 10

Duncan, I. D. (1992) *Guidelines for Clinical Practice and Programme Management,* NHS Cervical Screening Programme National Co-ordinating Network, Oxford.

Richart, R. M. (1990) A modified terminology for cervical intraepithelial neoplasia. *Obstet. Gynecol.,* **75**, 131–133.

Royal College of Obstetricians and Gynaecologists (1987) *Report of the Intercollegiate Working Party on Cervical Screening,* RCOG, London.

CHAPTER 12

Duncan, I. D. (1992) *Guidelines for Clinical Practice and Programme Management,* NHS Cervical Screening Programme National Co-ordinating Network, Oxford.

Kitchener, H. C., Cruickshank, M. C. and Farmery, E. (1995) The 1993 BSCCP/NCN United Kingdom Colposcopy Survey: comparison with 1988 and the response to introduction of guidelines. *Br. J. Obstet. Gynaecol.,* in press.

Lopes, A., Mor Yosef, S., Pearson, S. *et al.* (1990) Is routine colposcopic assessment necessary following laser ablation of cervical intraepithelial neoplasia? *Br. J. Obstet. Gynaecol.,* **97**, 175–177.

Paraskevaidis, E., Jandial, L., Mann E. *et al.* (1991) Pattern of treatment failure following laser for cervical intraepithelial neoplasia: implications for follow-up. *Obstet. Gynecol.,* **78**, 883.

CHAPTER 13

Nahhas, W., Sharkey, F. and Whitney, C. (1983) The prognostic significance of vascular channel involvement in deep stromal penetration in early cervical carcinoma. *Am. J. Clin. Oncol.,* **6**, 259.

Shingleton, H. M., Gore, H., Bradley, D. H. and Soong, S.-J. (1981) Adenocarcinoma of the cervix. I: Clinical evaluation and pathological features. *Am. J. Obstet. Gynecol.,* **139**, 799.

Van Nagell, J. Jr, Greenwell, N., Powell, D. and Donaldson, E. (1983) Microinvasive carcinoma of the cervix. *Am. J. Obstet. Gynecol.,* **145**, 981.

CHAPTER 16

Moss, T. and Hicks, D. A. (1994) *The Role of Genito-urinary Medicine Cytology and Colposcopy in Cervical Screening.* NHS Cervical Screening Programme: definitive document.

Paavonen, J., Stevens, C. E., Wølner-Hanssen, P. *et al.* (1988) Colposcopic manifestations of cervical and vaginal infections. *Obstet. Gynaecol. Survey,* **43**(7), 373–381.

CHAPTER 17

Chomet, J. and Chomet, J. (1989) *Cervical Cancer*, Thorsons, London.

Marteau, T., Walker, P., Giles, J. and Smail, M. (1990) *Br. J. Obstet. Gynaecol.,* **97**, 859–861.

Quilliam, S. (1989) *Positive Smear*, Penguin, Harmondsworth.

Index

Page numbers appearing in **bold** refer to figures.